Reviews and critical articles covering the entire field of normal anatomy (cytology, histology, cyto- and histochemistry, electron microscopy, macroscopy, experimental morphology and embryology and comparative anatomy) are published in Advances in Anatomy, Embryology and Cell Biology. Papers dealing with anthropology and clinical morphology that aim to encourage cooperation between anatomy and related disciplines will also be accepted. Papers are normally commissioned. Original papers and communications may be submitted and will be considered for publication provided they meet the requirements of a review article and thus fit into the scope of "Advances". English language is preferred.

It is a fundamental condition that submitted manuscripts have not been and will not simultaneously be submitted or published elsewhere. With the acceptance of a manuscript for publication, the publisher acquires full and exclusive copyright for all languages and countries.

Twenty-five copies of each paper are supplied free of charge.

Manuscripts should be addressed to

Co-ordinating Editor

Prof. Dr. H.-W. **KORF**, Zentrum der Morphologie, Universität Frankfurt, Theodor-Stern Kai 7, 60595 Frankfurt/Main, Germany
e-mail: korf@em.uni-frankfurt.de

Editors

Prof. Dr. F. **BECK**, Howard Florey Institute, University of Melbourne, Parkville, 3000 Melbourne, Victoria, Australia
e-mail: fb22@le.ac.uk

Prof. Dr. F. **CLASCÁ**, Department of Anatomy, Histology and Neurobiology,
Universidad Autónoma de Madrid, Ave. Arzobispo Morcillo s/n, 28029 Madrid, Spain
e-mail: francisco.clasca@uam.es

Prof. Dr. M. **FROTSCHER**, Institut für Anatomie und Zellbiologie, Abteilung für Neuroanatomie,
Albert-Ludwigs-Universität Freiburg, Albertstr. 17, 79001 Freiburg, Germany
e-mail: michael.frotscher@anat.uni-freiburg.de

Prof. Dr. D.E. **HAINES**, Ph.D., Department of Anatomy, The University of Mississippi Med. Ctr.,
2500 North State Street, Jackson, MS 39216-4505, USA
e-mail: dhaines@anatomy.umsmed.edu

Prof. Dr. N. **HIROKAWA**, Department of Cell Biology and Anatomy, University of Tokyo,
Hongo 7-3-1, 113-0033 Tokyo, Japan
e-mail: hirokawa@m.u-tokyo.ac.jp

Dr. Z. **KMIEC**, Department of Histology and Immunology, Medical University of Gdansk,
Debinki 1, 80-211 Gdansk, Poland
e-mail: zkmiec@amg.gda.pl

Prof. Dr. E. **MARANI**, Department Biomedical Signal and Systems, University Twente,
P.O. Box 217, 7500 AE Enschede, The Netherlands
e-mail: e.marani@utwente.nl

Prof. Dr. R. **PUTZ**, Anatomische Anstalt der Universität München,
Lehrstuhl Anatomie I, Pettenkoferstr. 11, 80336 München, Germany
e-mail: reinhard.putz@med.uni-muenchen.de

Prof. Dr. J.-P. **TIMMERMANS**, Department of Veterinary Sciences, University
Groenenborgerlaan 171, 2020 Antwerpen, Belgium
e-mail: jean-pierre.timmermans@ua.ac.be

205
Advances in Anatomy, Embryology and Cell Biology

Co-ordinating Editor

H.-W. Korf, Frankfurt

Editors

F. Beck, Melbourne · F. Clascá, Madrid
M. Frotscher, Freiburg · D.E. Haines, Jackson
N. Hirokawa, Tokyo · Z. Kmiec, Gdansk
E. Marani, Enschede · R. Putz, München
J.-P. Timmermans, Antwerpen

Michail S. Davidoff, Ralf Middendorff,
Dieter Müller,
Adolf F. Holstein

The Neuroendocrine Leydig Cells and their Stem Cell Progenitors, the Pericytes

With 22 Figures

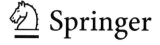

Michail S. Davidoff
University Medical Center
Hamburg-Eppendorf
Institute of Anatomy
Erika Haus, W29
Martinistr. 52
D-20246 Hamburg
Germany
e-mail: davidoff@uke.uni-hamburg.de

Dieter Müller
Justus-Liebig-University
Institute of Anatomy and Cell Biology
Aulweg 123
D-35385 Giessen
Germany
e-mail: hans-dieter.mueller@anatomie.med.uni-giessen.de

Ralf Middendorff
Justus-Liebig-University
Institute of Anatomy and Cell Biology
Aulweg 123
D-35385 Giessen
Germany
e-mail: ralf.middendorff@anatomie.med.uni-giessen.de

Adolf F. Holstein
University Medical Center
Hamburg-Eppendorf
Erika Haus, W29
Martinistr. 52
D-20246 Hamburg
Germany
e-mail: holstein@uke.uni-hamburg.de

ISSN 0301-5556
ISBN 978-3-642-00512-1   e-ISBN 978-3-642-00513-8
DOI 10.1007/978-3-642-00513-8
Springer Dordrecht Heidelberg London New York

Library of Congress Control Number: Applied for

© 2009 Springer-Verlag Berlin Heidelberg
This work is subject to copyright. All rights are reserved, whether the whole or part of the material is concerned, specifically the rights of translation, reprinting, reuse of illustrations, recitation, broadcasting reproduction on microfilm or in any other way, and storage in data banks. Duplication of this publication or parts thereof is permitted only under the provisions of the German Copyright Law of September 9, 1965, in its current version, and permission for use must always be obtained from Springer-Verlag. Violations are liable to prosecution under the German Copyright Law.
The use of general descriptive names, registered names, trademarks, etc. in this publication does not imply, even in the absence of a specific statement, that such names are exempt from the relevant protective laws and regulations and therefore free for general use.
Product liability: The publishers cannot guarantee the accuracy of any information about dosage and application contained in this book. In every individual case the user must check such information by consulting the relevant literature.

Printed on acid-free paper

Springer is part of Springer Science+Business Media (www.springer.com)

Acknowledgements

We are grateful to Theodor H. Schiebler, University of Würzburg, Germany, for initiation of this publication and useful suggestions, to Peter Kaufmann, Institute of Anatomy, Aachen, Germany, for interesting and helpful discussions, to Carl Schirren, Verein zur Förderung der Forschung auf dem Gebiete der Fortpflanzung e.V., Hamburg, for generous support of our work as well as to Freimut Leidenberger, formerly of the Institute for Hormone and Fertility Research, University of Hamburg, for kind co-operation. This work was in part supported by grants from the Deutsche Forschungsgemeinschaft (Ho 388/6-3; Ho 388/6-4; Da 459/1-1; Mi 637/1-1; Klinische Forschergruppe 181/1, project 4, to R.M.) and the Bundesminsterium für Bildung, Wissenschaft, Forschung und Technologie (BMBF), as part of a larger concerted project, "Fertilitätsstörungen" (01 KY 9502), and project 01 KY 9103/0 to D.M.

List of Contents

1	Introduction	1
2	**History of and Recent Progress in Leydig Cell Research**	3
2.1	More Than 150 Years Ago: The Discovery of Leydig Cells	3
2.2	100 Years Later: The Endocrine Characteristics of the Leydig Cells Were Revealed	5
2.3	Novel Aspects: Evidence for Neuroendocrine Properties of the Leydig Cells	6
2.4	Newer Results: Adult Leydig Cells Originate from Microvascular Mural Stem Cells (Pericytes and Vascular Smooth Muscle Cells)	8
3	**Morphology of the Leydig Cells**	9
3.1	Leydig Cells Represent a Heterogeneous Cell Population	9
4	**The Well-Known Endocrine Function of the Leydig Cells**	19
5	**The Neuroendocrine Properties of the Leydig Cells**	23
5.1	Considering Selected Substances	27
5.1.1	Neuronal Markers	27
5.1.2	Neuropeptides	28
5.1.3	γ-Aminobutyric acid	31
5.1.4	The NO/cGMP System	31
5.1.5	Neurotrophins and Their Receptors	33
5.1.6	Catecholamines	34
5.2	Hormones	36
5.2.1	Melatonin	38
5.3	Natriuretic Peptides	38
5.4	Neurofilament and Other Proteins	39
5.5	Astrocyte and Oligodendrocyte Marker Molecules	39
5.6	The Renin-Angiotensin System	40
5.7	VEGFs and Their Receptors	41
5.8	PDGFs and Their Receptors	42
6	**Development of the Testis**	45
6.1	The Testis Arises from the Urogenital Ridge and the Indifferent Gonad Rudiment	45
6.2	Primordial Germ Cells Migrate from the Epiblast into the Genital Ridges	45

6.3	The Sertoli Cells Emerge from Migrating Cells of the Coelomic Epithelium and Contribute to the Formation of the Testicular Cords	46
6.4	Migrating Mesonephric Cells Contribute to the Generation of Other Somatic Cells in the Male Gonad	47
7	**Development of the Neuroendocrine Leydig Cells.**	**49**
7.1	Two Main Leydig Cell Types Differentiate During Testis Development: The Fetal-Type and the Adult-Type Leydig Cells	49
7.2	Origin and Differentiation of the Adult Neuroendocrine Leydig Cells.	50
7.3	Definition and Classification of the Stem Cells	51
7.3.1	Embryonic Stem Cells	52
7.3.2	Fetal Stem Cells	52
7.3.3	Adult Stem Cells	52
7.4	Postnatal Development of the Neuroendocrine Leydig Cells in Rat and Mouse Testis.	53
7.4.1	New Data Concerning the Stem/Progenitor Cells of the Adult Leydig Cell Lineage.	53
7.4.2	Young Leydig Cells Are Surrounded by Basement Membrane Fragments, Supporting Their Origin from Perivascular Pericytes	67
7.4.3	Fetal-Like and Single-Spindle-Like Leydig Cells Are the First Leydig Cells That Appear During the Regeneration Process After EDS Administration in the Adult Rat Testis	67
7.4.4	Environmental Influences Are Responsible for the Diversity of Leydig Cell Phenotypes.	68
7.5	EDS Treatment of Adult Rats Also Leads To Damage of the Seminiferous Epithelium	69
7.6	The Pericyte Is a Peculiar Cell Type Just Now Beginning To Be Understood.	70
7.6.1	Pericytes and Vascular Smooth Muscle Cells Are of the Same Cell Lineage	70
7.6.2	Several Marker Antigens Characterize Pericytes and Smooth Muscle Cells of the Adult Rat Testis Microvasculature	71
7.6.3	Pericytes Are Stem/Progenitor Cells	72
7.6.4	Pericytes and Multipotent Mesenchymal Stem/Stromal Cells in Diverse Human and Rodent Tissues Comprise Mural and Perivascular Cells	73
7.6.5	Mesenchymal/Stromal Stem Cells Possess Remarkable Plasticity	78
7.7	The Vascular Stem Cell Niche and the Stem-Cell-Like Progenitors of Testicular Leydig Cells.	80
7.8	Leydig Cells May Be Continuously Generated from Stem/Progenitors Cells in the Testes of Adult Mammals	82
7.9	Postnatal Development of Leydig Cells in Rodent Testis	84
7.10	Postnatal Development of Leydig Cells in the Human Testis.	87
8	**Fetal and Adult Leydig Cells Are of Common Origin**	**89**
8.1	Where Do the Leydig Cell Ancestors Come from?	90
8.2	The Development of the Fetal Leydig Cells Is Closely Associated with the Development of the Testis Vasculature.	91
8.3	Leydig Cells, Blood Vessels and the Developing Testis	92
8.4	Are Stem Cells Really a Very Rare Population?	95
8.5	Leydig Stem/Progenitor Cells and the Neural Crest	98

8.5.1	Are Pericytes and Leydig Cells of Neuroectodermal/ Neural Crest Origin?...	98
8.5.2	Differences Between Neural Crest Cells from Head and Trunk Regions	101
8.5.3	The Potential Neural Crest Origin of the Leydig Cells and the Restricted Experimental Applicability of LacZ Transgenic Mice	102
8.6	The Aorta–Gonad–Mesonephros Region Harbours Many Diverse Stem Cells	102
9	**Concluding Remarks**...	105
References		109
Index		151

Chapter 1
Introduction

The Leydig cells of the testis were discovered more than 150 years ago, and 100 years later these cells were characterized as endocrine cells, which represent the main source of androgens. Androgens (testosterone and its metabolites) are of special importance for the development of the male reproductive tract, the development of male germ cells, the emergence of male secondary sex characteristics, the establishment of the hypothalamus-hypophysis-testis axis as well as the development of a male-specific structural differentiation of the brain. The idea of Leydig cells as endocrine cells has been the leading characteristic of this interesting cell population until now.

Many years after discovery of the endocrine nature of Leydig cells, numerous scientists found that biologically active substances other than testosterone are produced by Leydig cells and that these molecules are involved in the regulation of steroidogenesis and the communication among different testicular cell types. In this way, it became evident that in addition to the well-established control by steroids and systemic hormones, important local autocrine and paracrine control mechanisms of testicular functions exist. In this context, our studies over the last two decades allowed us to reveal a new important feature of Leydig cells, that is their obvious similarity to structures of the central and peripheral nervous system. This includes the expression of neurohormones, neurotransmitters, neuropeptides and glial cell antigens. These findings gave rise to the hypothesis of a potential neuroectodermal and/or neural crest origin of testicular Leydig cells. Recently, this idea was confirmed by data suggesting a relationship of Leydig cell stem/progenitors with cells of the epiblast, neuroectoderm and the neural crest.

Until now, the exact origin of Leydig cells is still a matter of debate. Most authors have suggested a mesenchymal origin. However, mesenchymal cells are descendants of all germinal layers. Thus, the term "mesenchymal origin" does not reflect a detailed description of the origin of Leydig cells, and the idea that Leydig cells are of multiple origin has been propagated up to the present. In this context, a large number of conflicting results has been published regarding the cells, the sites and the time of Leydig cell origin as well as the definition of the progeny of the Leydig stem/progenitor cells. Our discovery of neuroendocrine properties of Leydig stem/progenitor cells led to a new approach in the search for the Leydig stem/progenitor cells, and the testicular localization of the intermediate filament protein nestin, known to be expressed in neural stem cells, by our group was the first step to define mural cells (pericytes and vascular smooth muscle cells) of the testis microvasculature as the stem/progenitor cells of the adult Leydig cells. In summary, we were able to demonstrate specific proliferation of vascular progenitors and their subsequent transdifferentiation into steroidogenic Leydig cells, which – in addition – rapidly acquire neuronal and glial properties. Since both newly developed fetal and adult Leydig cell populations show the same features, a common origin of both populations seems likely.

Pericytes are distributed throughout the body, and there is convincing evidence for their stem/progenitor cell properties in diverse organs. Under appropriate (locally defined) conditions these pericytes, which reside in the vascular stem cell niche as dormant stem cells, become activated, proliferate, migrate and differentiate towards different somatic cell types of the body. Since most mesenchymal stem/progenitor cell types exhibit essential similarity to pericytes and certain mesenchymal stem cells represent pericyte descendants, we propose that mesenchymal stem cells in the perivascular niche are daughter cells of pericytes. Thus, pericytes are promising candidates for ancestor cells of all adult stem cells in the organism. There is strong evidence that early stem cells (cells arising during embryogenesis), such as the pericytes, exhibit both mesodermal and neural progeny, which might explain the neuroendocrine properties of the Leydig cells.

In this monograph, in addition to the description of some classical features of Leydig cells, we provide concise information on new features of Leydig cells, their origin and their relationship with the pericytes as their stem/progenitor cells. We mainly focus on the neuroendocrine characteristics of Leydig cells, their close association with testis vasculature, the transdifferentiation of their ancestors (the pericytes and smooth muscle cells) into fetal and young (blast, progenitor) Leydig cells and the role of pericytes as adult stem cells throughout the body.

Chapter 2
History of and Recent Progress in Leydig Cell Research

There are several comprehensive surveys on the history of the Leydig cells (see Christensen 1996, 2007, for reviews). Here we only provide some basic information on the initial discovery of this cell type. In addition, we specifically address those research results obtained during the subsequent course of research that are related to the identification of the endocrine and neuroendocrine properties of the Leydig cells and the striking interrelation between these cells and the testicular blood vessels.

2.1
More Than 150 Years Ago: The Discovery of Leydig Cells

The discovery of the Leydig cells was accompanied by some controversies. As noted by Hanes (1911), several authors (von Lenhossèk 1897; Plato 1896; Reinke 1896; Bouin and Ancel 1903) initially attributed the priority of the discovery of the interstitial cells of the testes to Kölliker (1854) instead of to Leydig (1850). However, Kölliker never insisted on being the person who discovered these cells, and in fact it was Leydig who for the first time (in 1850) reported on a new cell population situated within the interstitial space of the testes of some mammals (cf. Hanes 1911).

Leydig (1850) described these new cells as round, but he also detected single elongated cells within the intertubular area of the testes. Very importantly, already in this first description, Leydig (1850) recognized a narrow relationship between the interstitial cells and the testicular blood capillaries. Small aggregates of interstitial cells were frequently visible along blood vessels of the testicular intertubular space. If the interstitial cells were abundant, they were also found in a peritubular position. Also Henle (1866) described the fine granular Leydig cells as located in the neighbourhood of and along the testicular blood vessels, and he recognized that testicular blood vessels pass through the interstitial cell aggregates. Beissner (1898) reported on a contribution by Boll (1869, 1871) indicating that the Leydig cells form epithelial sheets or rows around testicular blood capillaries. In later publications, Waldeyer (1870, 1872) defined the interstitial cells of the testis as "perithelial" cells surrounding small testicular arteries. According to Waldeyer, the interstitial cells belong to the "embryonic cells of connective tissue". In contrast, Hofmeister (1872) claimed that the Leydig cells represent epithelial tissue which is independent of the course of the blood vessels within the intertubular space, since he did not observe direct contacts between these structures. Von Mihalkowitcs (1873) recognized within the intertubular space lymphatic vessels as well, but he noticed that the interstitial cells form a continuous and closed sheet around the testicular blood vessels (see also Henle 1866). Nussbaum (1880) reported that the interstitial substance in mammals, reptiles and birds follows the course of the testicular blood vessels. He also noted that the interstitial cells and the vessels do not have direct contacts but are separated by thin layers of connective tissue. According to Beissner (1898), the interstitial cells have no interrelation with the lamina propria and the blood vessels. He described that the covering membrane of the Leydig cells and the adventitia of the blood vessels are always separated by a distinct cleft. During a study of the ontogenic development of the testis of cats, Plato (1897) established that most of the interstitial cells were situated beneath the tunica albuginea (testicular capsule) in the vicinity of capillaries. Interestingly, he found only one mitotic figure in the typical interstitial cells. Von Ebner (1871) described interstitial cells as being located in the neighbourhood of blood vessels and that these cells do not have direct contact with the blood vessels. Jacobson (1879) provided a detailed description of the relationship between the interstitial cells and the testicular vessels. He reported that a larger number of Leydig cells could be seen at the branching point of the blood vessels. However, he also found numerous aggregates and single cells which were situated away from blood vessels, and he stated that the designation "perivascular tissue" (see Waldeyer 1870, 1872) is only partially compatible with the distribution variability of interstitial cell groups. All these early results concerning the relationship of the Leydig cells and the testicular blood vessels have to be interpreted with caution because the scientists had not examined serial sections and, in addition, they were not always able at that time to recognize the thin processes of the Leydig cells which remain in contact with the blood vessel wall even when their cell body lies separated in the vicinity of a capillary.

In the human testis, the interstitial cells were described for the first time by Kölliker (1854). Kölliker presumed that these cells resemble embryonic connective tissue cells (see also von Ebner 1871; von Hansemann 1895; Whitehead 1904). Furthermore, Kölliker for the first time reported that these cells are detectable in locations other than the interstitium, such as within the mediastinum, in the connective tissue septa and beneath the tunica albuginea (the capsule) of the testis, thus thereby providing the first information for the existence of ectopically (heterotopic) situated Leydig cells (see Jacobson 1879). In a later work, Henle (1866) did not agree with Kölliker's assumption that the interstitial cells are of connective tissue nature. In this respect, another opinion was presented by Hofmeister (1872), namely that the interstitial cells represent epithelial structures.

In some of these early Leydig cell studies, observations indicating a great variability between different species as well as within the same individual were made (Hoffmeister 1872). Moreover, Hoffmeister also for the first time reported on alterations in the number of Leydig cells during development. He recognized a reduced cell number during the late fetal development and an increase with the onset of puberty. In the testis of a 4-month-old boy, he found that the interstitial substance comprised two thirds of the testicular parenchyma volume, as compared with one tenth in an 8-month-old boy. During sexual maturity, the interstitial substance became enlarged, and in a 21-year-old man it was strongly developed and contained a large quantity of fat and pigment. Arrest of spermatogenesis and disappearance of the existing Leydig cell population during the hibernating period in marmot and its recovery in the spring was observed by von Hansemann (1895). The same author, in addition, reported the interesting findings that in patients suffering from some severe diseases, the germ cells disappeared, whereas the Leydig cells increased in number, providing the first evidence for the stability and to some extent the autonomy of the Leydig cell population in the testes. Similar results were reported later by Whitehead (1904), who, in addition, was able to observe a compensatory hypertrophy of the interstitial cells in the remaining contralateral testis of a pig in which one testis had been removed at an early age.

2.2
100 Years Later: The Endocrine Characteristics of the Leydig Cells Were Revealed

For a long time the functional significance of the Leydig cells remained undiscovered and a matter of debate. An interesting presumption, but without any significant experimental evidence, was that of Harvey (1875), who believed that the interstitial cells represent nerve cells. A secretory activity of the testes was hypothesized earlier by Berthold (1849 a,b), who showed that the loss of comb size and crowing in castrated rosters may be reversed by autotransplantation of testes. In human Leydig cells, special forms of protein-containing crystals were found within cytoplasm (Reinke 1896), later termed "crystals of Reinke". Reinke suggested that the presence of the crystals should indicate the ability of the interstitial cells to produce secretions (cf. Regaud and Policard 1901). Later, Bouin and Ancel (1903, 1904) studied normal and cryptorchid testes from various mammalian species and concluded that the interstitial cells are gland cells which as a whole represent a glandular organ, "la glande interstitielle". These cells were thought to be responsible for internal secretion and some additional trophic functions related to the germ cells and the Sertoli cells, providing the first idea for a possible regulatory role of the Leydig cells in the testes. The masculinizing factor, testosterone, was discovered firstly by David (1935) and David et al. (1935) in bovine testis. However, the first direct evidence that the Leydig cells of the testis are the producers of the male androgens was provided by Wattenberg (1958), who showed by histochemical techniques 3ß-hydroxysteroid dehydrogenase enzyme activity in the Leydig cells of the rabbit testis (see Christensen 1996, 2007). Some years later, Christensen (1965) and Christensen and Mason (1965) provided the first biochemical evidence for androgen synthesis by the cells of the interstitial tissue of the testes (see Hall et al. 1969; Neaves 1975).

The "classical" view regards the Leydig cells as the main source of production of androgens known to be important for the development of the male genital tract, the emergence of male secondary sex characteristics, the establishment of the hypothalamus-hypophysis-testis axis (see below), the structural differentiation of the male brain, resulting in a typical male behaviour, as well as for the processing and maintenance of steroidogenesis and spermatogenesis in the testis (Jégou and Pineau 1995; Ge et al. 1996). According to this view, testosterone synthesis and release are controlled by hypophyseal luteinizing hormone (LH) [or by placental human chorionic gonadotropin (hCG) during development]. Both hormones act via specific LH/hCG receptors, the second messenger cyclic adenosine monophosphate and protein kinase A. Testosterone released into the circulation inhibits by a feedback mechanism the expression of gonadotropin-releasing hormone in the hypothalamus, resulting in the cessation of LH secretion in the pituitary. In addition, testosterone directly inhibits the expression of LH in the pituitary gland. Thus, the regulatory circuit of androgen secretion ("hypothalamus-hypophysis-testis axis") comprises activities associated with the hypothalamus, the pituitary and the testis, respectively (for reviews, see Cooke et al. 1992; Weinbauer and Nieschlag 1995).

2.3
Novel Aspects: Evidence for Neuroendocrine Properties of the Leydig Cells

After the initial discovery of the endocrine nature of the Leydig cells, a lot of studies revealed that biologically active substances other than testosterone are locally produced within Leydig cells which are involved in the regulation of steroidogenesis and in the communication between testicular cells (Saez et al. 1995; Huhtaniemi and Toppari 1995; Jégou and Pineau 1995; Saez and Lejeune 1996). From this, it became evident that in addition to the classical control by systemic hormones and steroids, important local control mechanisms of testicular functions exist (de Kretser 1982, 1987; Kerr and Donachie 1986; Parvinen 1982; Sharpe 1983; Sharpe and Cooper 1987; Skinner and Fritz 1986; Verhoeven and Cailleau 1987). Among these substances, proopiomelanocortin (POMC)-derived peptides, such as adrenocorticotropic hormone, melanocyte-stimulating hormone, ß-endorphin (Bardin et al. 1987; Chen et al. 1984; Margioris et al. 1983; Tsong et al. 1982) and methionine-enkephalin (Met-Enk) were detected in Leydig cells of the rat testis (Saint-Pol et al. 1986), and it was suggested that these peptides contribute, by acting in a paracrine and/or an autocrine manner, to the regulation of testicular functions (Fabbri et al. 1988; Shaha et al. 1984). Although POMC derivatives were also found in other cell types and organs, these studies were the first to identify neuroactive substances in mammalian Leydig cells. However, the relationship between the Leydig cells and structures of the nervous system was not recognized at that time.

Based on and promoted by an extensive experience in research regarding the morphology and histochemistry of the nervous system, in 1985, our group started an investigation with the aim to examine whether human Leydig cells are immunoreactive for the opioid peptide Met-Enk. At the same time it was established that a large number of biologically active substances other than the "classical" neurotransmitters are expressed in different neuronal populations within the central and peripheral nervous system (Davidoff 1986; Gibson and Polak 1986; Hökfelt et al. 1980; Roberts and Allen 1986). Depending on the kind of its release and the mode of interaction with target cells, a neuroactive substance may act as a hormone, neurotransmitter or neuromodulator. One of these substances, a member of the tachykinin family, the undecapeptide substance P (SP), was found to be associated with primary afferent neurons and to play an important role in the processing of autonomic and somatic sensory (nociceptive) information in the central and peripheral nervous system (De Groat et al. 1983). Since opioid peptides had been detected in a number of different organs (Zagon et al. 1986), we additionally examined the possible localization in the testis of a neuropeptide (SP) confined at that time to neural structures only. In this case, we expected to see SP immunoreactivity in nerve fibres located in the vicinity of Leydig cells. These studies revealed that Met-Enk immunoreactivity, as demonstrated in the rat (Saint-Pol et al. 1986), is localized to human Leydig cells. However, we failed to find any SP immunoreactivity in nerve fibres. Instead, we detected SP immunoreactivity within the cytoplasm of the Leydig cells, with distinct differences in the staining intensity between individual cells. This investigation for the first time established that a substance, previously found exclusively in structures developmentally related to the nervous system, is expressed in "non-neuronal" human Leydig cells (Schulze et al. 1987 a, b; see Debeljuk et al. 2003 for a review). Consequently, these results raised two interesting questions regarding (1) whether Leydig cells are characterized by neuroendocrine properties and (2) whether this cell type is of a neuroectodermal origin (Schulze et al. 1987a; Davidoff et al. 1993).

By subsequent immunocytochemical studies, we were able to detect in human Leydig cells two additional neuroactive substances, namely the neuron-specific enolase (Schulze et al. 1991; Angelova et al. 1991c) and growth-associated protein-43, or neuromodulin (Davidoff et al. 1996).

On the basis of these initial findings but taking into account (1) that certain neuronal markers may also appear in non-neuronal cell types and (2) that the demonstration of a marker substance by itself cannot in general be accepted as sufficient evidence for the neuroendocrine phenotype of a cell, we started a lot of additional studies to investigate potential neuroendocrine properties of the Leydig cells. At the beginning, we established that the expression of neuropeptides in human Leydig cells is not a species-specific phenomenon. By these studies, we found that SP, neuron specific enolase and Met-Enk immunoreactivities are also detectable in Leydig cells of other species such as mouse, rat, hamster,and guinea pig (Angelova and Davidoff 1989; Angelova et al. 1991a, b), although certain species-related differences became evident.

In the following years, we found immunoreactivity for a great number of neural and glial markers in Leydig cells (Davidoff et al. 2001, 2002). By electron microscopy, we detected in human Leydig cells distinct clear and dense-core vesicles, potentially related to the established synaptophysin and chromogranin A immunoreactivity (Davidoff et al. 1996). Taken together, these results revealed that human and animal Leydig cells share great similarity to cells of the diffuse neuroendocrine system (Pearse 1969, 1986) or to paraneurons (Fujita 1989) (see also Schulze et al. 1987a; Angelova et al. 1991a-c). In 1993, the cumulative arguments indicating the neuroendocrine nature of Leydig cells were outlined (Davidoff et al. 1993). In this context, it is important to note that the neuroendocrine phenotype of Leydig cells remains largely conserved even after disturbances of testicular functions (Middendorff et al. 1993) or under conditions of Leydig cell hyperplasia and cancer (Middendorff et al. 1995).

2.4
Newer Results: Adult Leydig Cells Originate from Microvascular Mural Stem Cells (Pericytes and Vascular Smooth Muscle Cells)

The elucidation of the neuroendocrine nature of rodent and human Leydig cells provided the basis for the discovery of their stem/progenitor cells. By monitoring an experimentally induced, synchronized regeneration of a new Leydig cell population in adult rats, we were able to establish that Leydig cells originate from components (pericytes and vascular smooth muscle cells) of the testis microvasculature. Located within a vascular stem cell niche, they act as silencing adult stem cells. The progenitor (young, blast) Leydig cells arise from these ancestors by a process known as transdifferentiation (see Chaps. 7-9).

Chapter 3
Morphology of the Leydig Cells

3.1
Leydig Cells Represent a Heterogeneous Cell Population

Several updated reviews on the Leydig cell structure (Russell 1996; Pudney 1996) and structural aspects related to Leydig cell development and functional activities have already been published (Chemes 1996; Pelliniemi et al. 1996; Ge et al. 1996; Haider 2004; Haider et al. 2007; Prince 2007). Here we will address only certain structural features that are characteristic for human and rodent Leydig cells.

The Leydig cells represent a heterogeneous cell population. There are significant differences in the organization, number, shape and other cellular properties of the Leydig cells between species (Pudney 1996; Russel 1996; Prince 2007). In addition to the species-related differences, peculiarities based on developmental, metabolic, functional and seasonal influences have to be considered (Callard 1996; Haider et al. 2007).

There exist a number of comprehensive reviews regarding structural and functional features of mammalian (including human) Leydig cells (Mancini et al. 1963; Nishimura and Kondo 1964; Christensen 1970, 1975; Kerr and de Kretser 1981; de Kretser and Kerr 1994; Schulze 1984). An updated characterization of human Leydig cells and a detailed description of their similarities/dissimilarities with regard to the Leydig cells of other species have been provided recently (Chemes 1996; Pudney 1996).

The Leydig cells of adult human testes show a pronounced morphological heterogeneity. This is especially true for the testes of elderly men and the testes of patients with reduced or impaired spermatogenesis (Schulze 1984; Chen et al. 1996b; Holstein and Roosen-Runge 1981; Holstein et al. 1988).

As is evident from light microscopy, human Leydig cells differ in size, and their morphological appearance ranges from polygonal, round, elongated to occasionally spindle-shaped cells. They usually contain excentric nuclei, which are round and distinguished by prominent nucleoli and peripherally distributed heterochromatin (Figs. 3.1, 3.2). Numerous dark-stained organelles and lipofuscin inclusions are

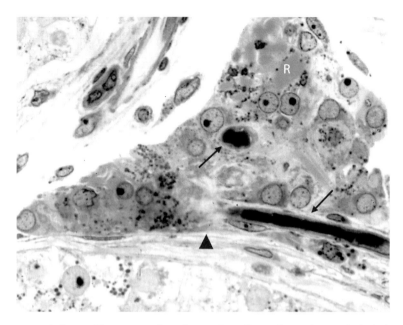

Fig. 3.1 Morphology of human Leydig cells. Leydig cells are located peritubularly (arrowhead) and around longitudinally (arrow) and horizontally (arrow) cut capillaries. Most of the Leydig cells exhibit a round nucleus with excentric nucleoli. Numerous densely stained granules in their cytoplasm represent different organelles and inclusions. Reinke cristalloids (R) are visible as homogenous grey fields in the cytoplasm. Semithin section, ×850

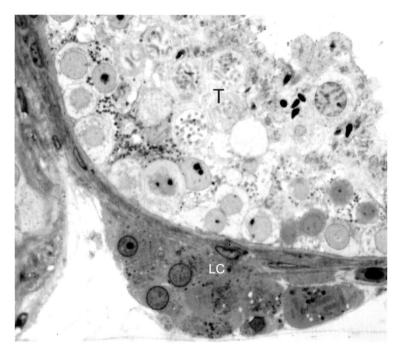

Fig. 3.2 Peritubular Leydig cells. A segment of a seminiferous tubule (T) and a peritubular group of large Leydig cells (LC) in the human testis are visible. Semithin section, ×850

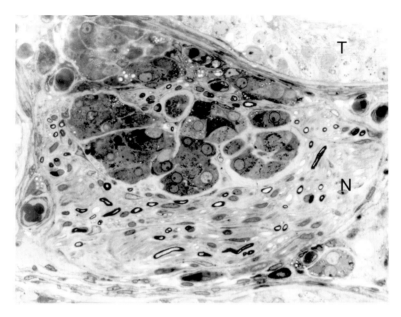

Fig. 3.3 Heterogeneous morphology of human Leydig cells. A group of polymorphic Leydig cells with different numbers of cytoplasmic organelles is visible between a tubule (T) and a peripheral nerve bundle (N). Semithin section, ×380

seen in the perinuclear region. The cytoplasm consists of relatively homogenous dark- and light-stained areas. Some cells contain Reinke crystalloids (Fig. 3.1), a structure found almost exclusively in human Leydig cells (Schulze 1984; Chemes 1996). Clusters of Leydig cells are intimately associated with bundles of peripheral nerves (Fig. 3.3).

Electron microscopically, human Leydig cells are seen distributed as single cells or as (small or larger) groups within the interstitial tissue, frequently in the vicinity or around blood vessels (Schulze 1984; Figs. 3.4, 3.5). Rarely, rows of Leydig cells, running parallel to the border of the lamina propria (peritubular Leydig cells; Fig. 3.5) or located within the lamina propria (Fig. 3.6; Schulze and Holstein 1978; Davidoff et al. 1990) are detectable. In the latter case, they frequently show a peripheral localization, near the outer sheath of connective tissue cells separating the lamina propria from the interstitial space (Schulze 1984; Holstein et al. 1996). Usually, individual Leydig cells or Leydig cell groups are surrounded by thin processes of "encapsulating fibroblasts" (Chemes 1996) or "compartmentalizing cells" (Co-cells) (Figs. 3.7, 3.8) which express substances normally found in glial cells of the central and peripheral nervous system (Holstein and Davidoff 1997). The surface of the Leydig cells is separated from the Co-cells by a sheath (of variable thickness) of extracellular matrix filaments (Figs. 3.7, 3.8). The Co-cells

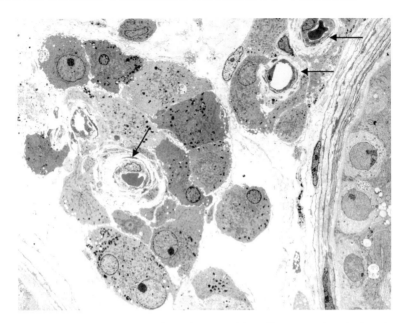

Fig. 3.4 Ultrastructure of human Leydig cells. Most of the cells surround testicular microvessels (arrows). Note the differences in density of Leydig cell cytoplasm and in organelle status. Electron micrograph, ×1,100

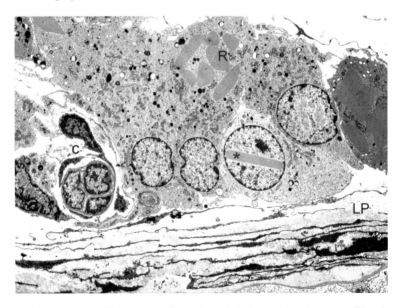

Fig. 3.5 Ultrastructure of human Leydig cells and their vicinity. A group of Leydig cells is visible in vicinity of a blood capillary (c) and the peritubular lamina propria (LP). Note Reinke crystalloids (R) within the cytoplasm of some Leydig cells and a paracrystalline structure (asterisk) in the nucleus of one cell. Electron micrograph, ×2,500

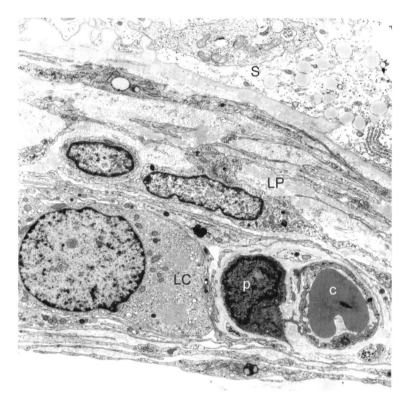

Fig. 3.6 Ultrastructure of a Leydig cell and an adjacent pericyte. A Leydig cell (LC) and a capillary (c) with a pericyte (p) are seen in the periphery of the lamina propria (LP) of a seminiferous tubule in human testis. S basal cytoplasm of a Sertoli cell. Electron micrograph, ×4,800

differ in the expression of several antigens depending on their (peritubular vs. interstitial) location (Holstein and Davidoff 1997).

On the basis of examinations by transmission electron microscopy, Leydig cells are distinguished by an abundance of smooth endoplasmic reticulum of varying (tubulovesicular, lamellar) arrangements. They also typically contain pleiomorphic (tubular and lamellar association forms) mitochondria as well as vesicles (also groups of dense-core vesicles) and lipid droplets of different size and density (Russel 1996; Schulze 1984; Chemes 1996; Prince 2007). Some of these cellular constituents are believed to be characteristic of steroidogenic cells (Fig. 3.3).In addition, human Leydig cells possess well-developed Golgi complexes and numerous lysosomes and lysosomal derivatives of varied morphology and size (Prince 2007). Varying numbers of lipofuscin granules, peroxisomes as well as crystalloid or paracrystalline structures other than the Reinke crystalloids (Figs. 3.5, 3.9, 3.10) could also

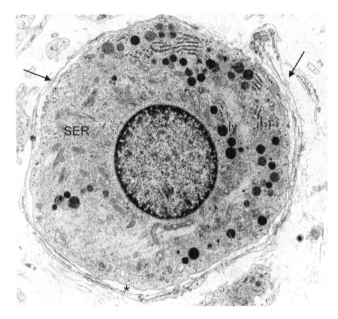

Fig. 3.7 Ultrastructure of a single round Leydig cell of the human testis. The cell is surrounded by thin compartmentalizing cells (arrows) found at different distances from the Leydig cell body and separated from it by a sheath of extracellular matrix filaments (asterisk). Note the abundance of smooth endoplasmic reticulum (SER), lysosomal-like (ly) structures and inclusions within the Leydig cell cytoplasm. Electron micrograph, ×5,500

be found within the cytoplasm and nucleus of the Leydig cells. In addition, rough endoplasmic reticulum, ribosomes and cytoskeletal components such as microtubules, actin and intermediate filaments belong to the detectable structural elements of the Leydig cells (Figs. 3.7, 3.8).

In testes of certain patients with reduced spermatogenesis, relatively small Leydig cells with cytoplasm processes of different length and sometimes secondary branches arise. These cells are found in the intertubular space in the form of small or large cell groups. Large polygonal or round Leydig cells are frequently located in their direct vicinity (Fig. 3.11). In the processes of these Leydig cells, intermediate filaments and a variety of cytoplasmic vesicles (Schulze 1984; Chemes 1996; Prince 2007) are characteristically distributed (Figs. 3.12–3.14). Between these processes and the body of adjacent Leydig cells (like between the plasma membranes of neighbouring Leydig cells), desmosome-like contacts and gap junctions (Figs. 3.13, 3.14) were established (Nagano and Suzuki 1976; Schulze 1984; Russell 1996;

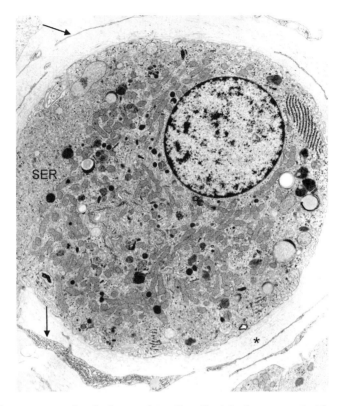

Fig. 3.8 Ultrastructure of a single round Leydig cell of the human testis. The cell is surrounded by thin compartmentalizing cells (arrows) found at different distances from the Leydig cell body and separated from it by a sheath of extracellular matrix filaments (asterisk). Note the abundance of smooth endoplasmic reticulum (SER), mitochondria, and inclusions within the cytoplasm. Electron micrograph, ×5,500

Chemes 1996; Prince 2007). In mouse and rat testes, gap junctions of the Leydig cells contain connexin 43 and carry signals that regulate their secretory activity (Perez-Armendariz et al. 1994).

Some typical features of Leydig cells are affected by developmental influences. For Leydig cells of the human testis, Prince (2007) defined three developmental periods: fetal, neonatal and adult, each associated with typical differences in the cellular ultrastructure. For example, Reinke crystalloids are present in adult Leydig cells but are absent in fetal and immature Leydig cells.

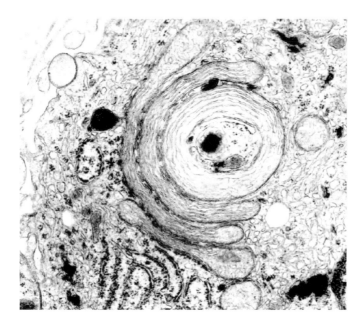

Fig. 3.9 Ultrastructure of cytoplasmic components of human Leydig cells. Concentric arrangements of the smooth endoplasmic reticulum. Electron micrograph, × 12,300

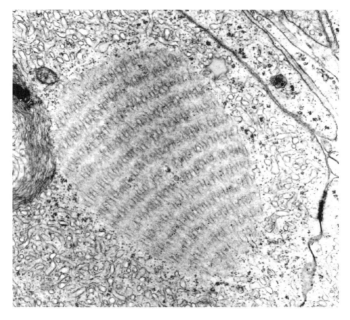

Fig. 3.10 Condensation of the reticulum in the form of an annulate lamella. Electron micrograph, ×11,000

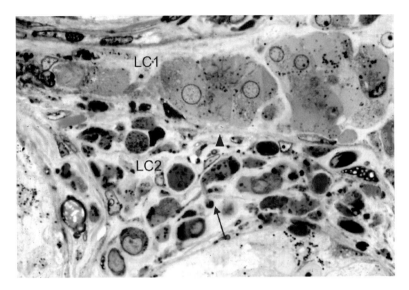

Fig. 3.11 Leydig cell groups of completely different phenotypes in close vicinity. Two Leydig cell groups separated by a thin layer of connective tissue (arrowhead) are visible. One group (LC1) consists of large round and polygonal Leydig cells with light cytoplasm. Another group (LC2) comprises smaller dark cells of different shape and form, some of which show partially branching processes with buttonlike enlargements (arrow). Semithin section, ×600

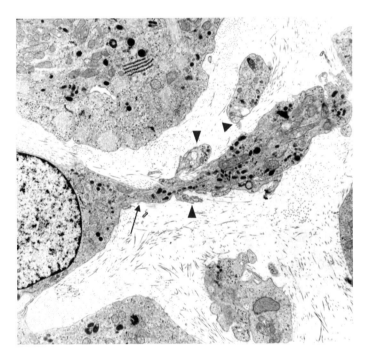

Fig. 3.12 Transmission electron micrograph of human Leydig cells with primary (arrow) and secondary (arrowhead) branching processes on longitudinal sections (×5,500)

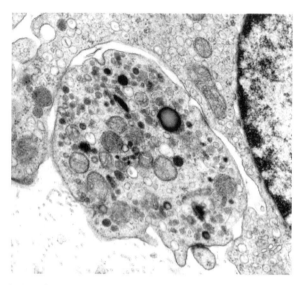

Fig. 3.13 Transmission electron micrograph of human Leydig cells. Note branching processes and the abundance of heterogeneous storage vesicles within the cytoplasm (×16,000)

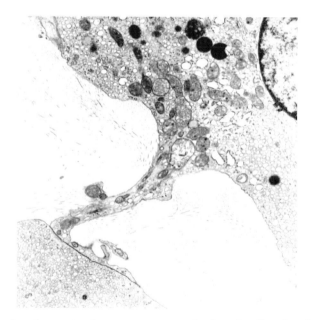

Fig. 3.14 A gap junction contact between an outgrowth of one Leydig cell and the cell body membrane of a neighbouring Leydig cell (×5,000)

Chapter 4
The Well-Known Endocrine Function of the Leydig Cells

Several reviews have addressed the biochemistry and possible functional significance of different agents in the developing and mature Leydig cells (Saez 1994; Russell 1996; Pelliniemi et al. 1996; Lejeune et al. 1998; Habert et al. 2001; Haider 2004).

Moreover, numerous publications have been devoted to the steroidogenic capacity of the Leydig cells in mammals and human (Chen et al. 1996b; Payne and O'Shaughnessy 1996; Haider 2004; Stocco 2007). There is no doubt that the Leydig cells represent the main cell type of the testis that is able to produce androgens from cholesterol (Christensen and Mason 1965; Hall et al. 1969; Bardin 1996; Freeman and Rommerts 1996; Payne and O'Shaughnessy 1996; Stocco 2007, for reviews). Several recent publications highlight the factors (hormones, growth factors, enzymes, receptors) involved in the production and metabolism of androgens (Chandrashekar and Bartke 2007; O'Shaughnessy et al. 2007a, b; Carreau 2007, 2008; Haider et al. 2007; Ge and Hardy 2007; Chen et al. 2007; Stocco 2007; Payne 2007). Leydig cells possess the molecular machinery necessary for binding and receptor-mediated endocytosis of low-density lipoproteins, de novo synthesis of cholesterol and its transport towards the mitochondria, where it will be converted to pregnenolone by cytochrome P450 side chain cleavage enzyme at the inner mitochondrial membrane. In the Leydig cells, the lipid droplets are storage sites of cholesterol esters. The transport of cholesterol from the outer to the inner mitochondrial membrane is a rate-limiting step and is mediated by steroidogenic acute regulatory protein (Stocco 2007). Three additional steps involving enzymes located in the Leydig cell cytoplasm lead to the formation of androgen precursors and biologically active androgens such as testosterone (Weinbauer and Nieschlag 1990; Saez 1994; Payne 2007). Leydig cells also contain the enzyme aromatase, which is implicated in the conversion of the C_{19} androgens androstenedione and testosterone to the C_{18} oestrogens oestrone and oestradiol (Carreau 2007, 2008; Payne 2007).

In Leydig cells of different species, enzymes involved in the synthesis and metabolism of steroids such as 3β-hydroxysteroid dehydrogenase (3β-HSD)/ Δ^5- Δ^4-isomerase, 17β-hydroxysteroid dehydrogenase, 11β-hydroxysteroid dehydrogenase, 5α-reductase as well as the testosterone produced (Bardin 1996; Dupont et al. 1993; Ge et al. 1996; Haider et al. 1986; Risbridger 1996; Saez 1994; Payne 2007) could be demonstrated by biochemical and/or immunological approaches. Testosterone-like immunoreactivity was detectable in human Leydig cells, located inter- or peritubularly as well as in cells residing within the tunica albuginea (Figs. 3.6-3.8).

In human Leydig cells, immunohistochemical staining for 3ß-HSD seems less pronounced than in rat Leydig cells. However, as is the case for testosterone, the immunoreactivity (Regadera et al. 1993) for 3ß-HSD activity varies considerably among individual patients. This is consistent with biochemical and clinical findings (Klinefelter and Kelce 1996; Swredloff and Wang 2007). Moreover, in Leydig cells of adjacent areas as well as among the Leydig cells within single clusters, differences in 3ß-HSD activity are seen, probably reflecting variations in the functional activity of individual Leydig cells and/or indicating phenotypic variants (see below).

Human Leydig cells exhibit immunoreactivity for low-density-lipoprotein receptors, consistent with the idea that they can bind and internalize exogenous cholesterol for further utilization in the steroidogenic process. Furthermore, in Leydig cells of the human testis, androgen receptors (ARs), oestrogen receptors and luteinizing hormone(LH)/human chorion gonadotropin (hCG) receptors are detectable immunocytochemically (see below).

The "classical" view considers the Leydig cells as the main source of production of androgens, with an important impact for development of the male genital tract, male secondary sex characteristics and behaviour as well as for the processing and maintenance of steroidogenesis and spermatogenesis in testis (Huhtaniemi and Toppari 1995). According to this view, testosterone synthesis and release are controlled by LH or placental hCG during development. Both hormones act via specific LH/hCG receptors, the second messenger cyclic adenosine monophosphate and protein kinase A activity (Dufau and Tsai-Morris 2007). Testosterone released into the blood circulation inhibits by a feedback mechanism the expression of gonadotropin-releasing hormone in the hypothalamus, resulting in the cessation of LH secretion in the pituitary gland. In addition, testosterone directly inhibits the expression of LH by the hypophysis. By this, the regulatory circuit of the androgen secretion, in which the hypothalamus, the hypophysis and the testis are involved, appears closed (Cooke et al. 1992; Weinbauer and Nieschlag 1995, for a review; Callard 1996). Recently, a brain and reproductive organ-expressed gene (BRE) was found in Leydig tumour cells (mLTC-1) to inhibit steroidogenesis by downregulating 3ß-HSD (Miao et al. 2005).

AR messenger RNA was detected in the cytoplasm of Leydig cells, pericytes, peritubular myoid and Sertoli cells (Shan et al. 1995a). Immunohistochemically, AR protein was detected in the nuclei of spindle-shaped Leydig cell progenitors at postnatal day 21, of immature Leydig cells at postnatal day 35 and of adult Leydig cells at postnatal day 90. Importantly, nuclear AR was also detected in pericytes or vascular smooth muscle cells, respectively (Bergh and Damber 1992; Bremner et al. 1994; Vornberger et al. 1994; Atanassova et al. 2006). In a recent study, De Gendt et al. (2005) investigated the generation of adult Leydig cells in mice with Sertoli-cell-selective or total ablation of the AR. The results revealed that elimination of androgen actions in Sertoli cells has major consequences for Leydig cell development and suggested that this could be mediated indirectly via platelet-derived growth factor A and/or oestrogens/oestrogen sulphotransferase (Sharpe et al. 2003). In addition, Shan et al. (1997) found that testosterone produced by Leydig cells has paracrine effects on Sertoli cells which are critical for the maintenance of spermatogenesis throughout adulthood. Leydig cell androgens also have autocrine effects in prepubertal rats by influencing early Leydig cell function and differentiation. Androgen inhibits testosterone production by adult Leydig cells but facilitates their pubertal differentiation (Hardy et al. 1990). In the absence of ARs, fetal Leydig cells are normal, but the maturation of adult Leydig cells is partially disturbed (O'Shaughnessy et al. 2002).

Mature Leydig cells may produce oestrogen acting as a paracrine factor controlling (inhibiting) precursor cell development and steroidogenesis of the adult Leydig cell population (Sharpe 1990; Abney and Myers 1991; O'Donnell et al. 2001). Atanassova et al. (1999) established that exposure of neonatal rats to oestrogen induced dose-dependent alterations in Sertoli cell number, germ cell volume, efficiency of spermatogenesis and germ cell apoptosis in adulthood. However, low levels of oestrogens can advance the first wave of spermatogenesis at puberty (Atanassova et al. 2000). As shown by Delbès et al. (2005), endogenous oestrogens inhibit steroidogenesis via oestrogen receptor α by acting directly on testes during early fetal and neonatal development.

Important for the elimination of oestrogen activity is oestrogen sulphotransferase, a cytosolic enzyme that catalyses the sulphoconjugation and inactivation of oestrogens. It is expressed abundantly in mammalian testes, where it may modulate the activity of locally produced oestrogen. Oestrogen sulphotransferase plays a physiological role in protecting Leydig cells from oestrogen-induced biochemical lesions and provides an example for regulation of tissue oestrogen sensitivity by proteins different from oestrogen receptors (Qian and Song 1999; Tong et al. 2004).

The C_{19} steroid dehydroepiandrosterone (DHEA) is produced after the cleavage of pregnenolone by testicular 17α-hydroxylase cytochrome P450 during steroidogenesis in testis (Payne 2007), where the enzyme is found in Leydig cells (Murray et al. 2000; Pelletier et al. 2001; Weng et al. 2005; Raeside et al. 2006). DHEA is also involved in the maintenance and division of human neural stem cells. DHEA is a neurosteroid with potential effects on neurogenesis and neuronal survival in humans. Suzuki et al. (2004) showed that DHEA significantly increased the growth rates of neural stem cells derived from the fetal cortex.

Chapter 5
The Neuroendocrine Properties of the Leydig Cells

The testis produces a lot of biologically active substances that are implicated in the local regulation of steroidogenesis and the communication between testicular cells (Schulze et al. 1987a, 1991; Risbridger 1996; Saez 1994; Klinefelter and Kelce 1996; Lejeune et al. 1998; Angelova et al. 1991a; Ciampani et al. 1992; Gnessi et al. 1992; Guldenaar and Pickering 1985; Ivell et al. 1990; Koike and Nomura 1993; Middendorff et al. 1993, 1995; Mayerhofer 1996; Mukhopadhyay et al. 1995; Murono et al. 1992; Tinajero et al. 1993a, b; Schumacher et al. 1992, 1993; Ungefroren et al. 1994). Examples include hormones such as arginine-vasopressin, oxytocin, gonadotropin-releasing hormone (GnRH), corticotropin-releasing hormone (CRH), follicle-stimulating hormone (FSH), prolactin, calcitonin, thyroid hormones, steroid hormones (androgens, oestrogens and glycocorticoids), growth factors and cytokines (basic fibroblast growth factor, FGF2; insulin-like growth factor I; inhibins; activins; transforming growth factor α, TGF-α; transforming growth factor β, TGF-ß; epidermal growth factor, EGF; platelet-derived growth factor, PDGF; interleukin-1), some Sertoli cell factors as well as neuronal transmitters and regulatory peptides (catecholamines; 5-hydroxytryptamine, 5-HT; melatonin; substance P, SP; proopiomelanocortin derivatives; natriuretic peptides; endothelins; angiotensin II; erythropoietin). They were shown to act through different second messengers or directly on enzymes responsible for the synthesis of androgens. Importantly, and indicating the neuroendocrine nature of the Leydig cells, a large number of the above-mentioned substances are expressed in postmitotic adult as well as in differentiating neurons or in glial cells of the nervous system.

In addition to demonstrating steroidogenic activity (3ß-hydroxysteroid dehydrogenase), low-density-lipoprotein receptor, testosterone, androgen receptor, oestrogen receptor as well as oestrogen receptor binding protein immunoreactivity, we were able to identify (Davidoff et al. 1996; unpublished results) a large number of substances with partially neuronal and neuroendocrine characteristics in human and some mammalian Leydig cells as listed below:

Neuronal markers

Neuron-specific enolase (NSE)
Growth-associated protein 43 (GAP-43), or neuromodulin

Neuronal nuclei (NeuN) antigen
Transcription factor neuroD$_1$ (NeuroD)
Protein gene product 9.5

Synaptic and storage vesicle proteins

Synaptophysin
Synaptic binding protein 25
Chromogranin A and chromogranin B

Cytoskeletal proteins

Neurofilament protein 200 (NF-H)
Neurofilament protein 160 (NF-M)
Neurofilament protein 68 (NF-L)
Microtubule-associated protein 2 (MAP-2)
Nestin

Cell adhesion molecules

Neural cell adhesion molecule (NCAM)
Human natural killer cell glycan
Pan cadherin

Indoleamines

5-Hydroxytryptamine (5-HT)
Tryptophan hydroxylase (TPH)

Enzymes involved in the synthesis of catecholamines

Tyrosine hydroxylase (TH)
Aromatic L-amino acid decarboxylase (AADC)
Dopamine ß-hydroxylase (DBH)
Phenylethanolamine N-methyltransferase (PNMT)

Neurohormones and/or their receptors

Growth-hormone-releasing hormone (GHRH)
Corticotropin-releasing hormone (CRH)
Luteinizing-hormone-releasing hormone (LHRH)
Luteinizing hormone receptor (LHR)
GnRH receptor

Neurotrophins and neurotrophin receptors

Nerve growth factor (NGF)
Neurotrophin-3 (NT-3)/neurotrophin-4 (NT-4)
Brain-derived neurotrophic factor (BDNF)
receptor p75^{NTR} (p75^{NTR})
Neurotrophin receptor TrkA
Neurotrophin receptor TrkB

Neurotrophin receptor TrkC
Glial cell line derived neurotrophic factor (GDNF)
GDNF receptors: GFRα-1 and GFRα-2

Neuropeptides and/or their receptors

SP
SP receptor
Neurokinin A
Neurokinin A receptor
Methionine-enkephalin
ß-Endorphin
Neurotensin
Neuropeptide tyrosine (NPY)
Vasoactive intestinal (poly) peptide (VIP)
Peptide histidine isoleucine
Atrial natriuretic peptide (ANP)
Brain natriuretic peptide (BNP)
C-type natriuretic peptide (CNP)
Big endothelin
Endothelin I
Endothelin II
Endothelin receptor type A
Endothelin receptor type B

Glial cell antigens

Galactocerebroside (GalC)
Cyclic 2,3-nucleotide 3′-phosphodiesterase (CNPase)
Glial fibrillary acidic protein (GFAP)
A2B5 antigen (A2B5)
O4 sulphatide (O4)

Calcium-binding proteins

Protein S-100 (S-100)
Calmodulin (CaM)
Calbindin-D28
Parvalbumin

Components of the nitric oxide (NO)/cyclic GMP (cGMP) system

NO synthase (NOS), brain type (NOS-1)
NOS, macrophage type (NOS-2)
NOS, endothelial type (NOS-3)
Soluble guanylyl cyclase (sGC)
cGMP
Aspartate
Glutamate

Calmodulin (CaM)
Ca^{2+}/CaM-dependent protein kinase II (Ca^{2+}/CaM PK II)
Superoxide dismutase

Components of the renin/angiotensin system

Prorenin
Renin
Angiotensin I
Angiotensin II
Angiotensin receptor type I

Growth factors and/or their receptors

Activin
Inhibin A
Transforming growth factor ß$_1$
TGF-α
Insulin-like growth factor I
Insulin-like growth factor II
Insulin-like growth factor binding proteins 1, 2, 3, 4, 5, 6
Insulin-like peptide 3
G protein coupled receptor 2 (RXFP2; previously LGR8)
Epidermal growth factor receptor
FGF2
Vascular endothelial growth factor (VEGF)
Vascular endothelial growth factor receptor (VEGFR)
Endothelial cell growth factor
Platelet-derived growth factor B (PDGF-B)
Platelet-derived growth factor B receptor (PDGFR-B)
Interleukins (interleukin-1α)
Macrophage growth factor

The expression of all these substances characterizes the Leydig cells of vertebrate testes as a cell population with at the same time endocrine (steroidogenic), neuroendocrine and glial cell features. We emphasize that the results obtained in our immunohistochemical studies were based on the application of highly effective amplification techniques which allowed the detection/visualization of very small quantities of a given substance on tissue sections of paraffin-embedded testicular material (Davidoff and Schulze 1990). This could explain, besides the occurrence of species-related differences, the failure to detect some of these antigens in other studies. Furthermore, the identification of a molecule, especially when present in a low quantity, does not necessarily indicate its functional activity in Leydig cells. In addition, the expression of such molecules may significantly change during different developmental stages of the Leydig cells. In any case, they should represent useful markers for the exact determination of the cell phenotype and the relation of the Leydig cells to other cell types of the organism. Although adult Leydig cells

5.1 Considering Selected Substances

In the following, we specifically address some of these molecules, with a focus on relationships between testicular Leydig cells and structures of the central and peripheral nervous system or the microvasculature.

5.1.1 Neuronal Markers

5.1.1.1 Neuron-Specific Enolase

NSE is a glycolytic enzyme nearly exclusively expressed in most differentiated neurons and neuroendocrine cells. NSE expression begins shortly after initiation of synaptogenesis. NSE was visualized by immunohistochemistry in (both developing and adult) human (Schulze et al. 1991; Sklebar et al. 2008), golden hamster, rat and guinea pig Leydig cells on tissue sections as well as in primary cultures of Leydig cells isolated from adult hamster testes (Angelova et al. 1991c). Interestingly, the staining intensity was different between fetal- and adult-type Leydig cells.

5.1.1.2 Growth-Associated Protein 43

In Leydig cells of the human testis, we were able to visualize GAP-43-like immunoreactivity. GAP-43 (B-50, neuromodulin) is a cytoplasmic protein implicated in axonal growth, neuronal differentiation, plasticity and regeneration. Its activities are regulated by dynamic interactions with various neuronal proteins, including actin and brain spectrin. There is evidence that GAP-43 colocalizes and potentially interacts with MAP-2 in adult and fetal rat brain, as well as in primary neuronal cultures. It is further suggested that this interaction may be developmentally regulated (Chakravarthy et al. 2008). GAP-43 is also expressed in multipotent precursors, and its absence affects the differentiation of both neurons and astrocytes of the central nervous system (Fujimori et al. 2008).

5.1.1.3 NeuN Antigen

Immunoreactivity for the NeuN antigen was well detectable in the cytoplasm of human Leydig cells. In the nervous system, NeuN is localized to nuclei of mature neurons and defines postmitotic neurons or differentiated neuronal precursors as well as nuclei of astrocytes. In western blots, it could be demonstrated as protein bands at 46 and 48 kDa, and as a minor band at 66 kDa (Darlington et al. 2008).

5.1.1.4
NeuroD

We found the human Leydig cells show in addition moderate immunoreactivity for the antigen neuroD. NeuroD is a transcription factor, representing a member of the basic helix-loop-helix protein family expressed in the central nervous system (Kamath et al. 2005). This factor plays an essential role in the terminal differentiation of neural progenitor cells, including astrocytes. NeuroD also regulates multiple functions in the developing neural retina such as neuron versus glial cell fate decision and interneuron development, and is essential for survival of a subset of rod photoreceptors (Morrow et al. 1999).

5.1.2
Neuropeptides

The neuropeptides play pivotal roles for the development, maturation and maintenance of neural structures. There are a vast number of reports providing unequivocal evidence that neuropeptides are important for the functional activity of neural stem and progenitor cells during early development of the nervous system. Neuropeptides, in addition, act as neurotransmitters or neuromodulators for the normal functioning of the adult central and peripheral nervous system.

5.1.2.1
Tachykinins

As mentioned already, the first neuronal transmitter substance revealed in Leydig cells was SP (Schulze et al. 1987a; Angelova and Davidoff 1989; Angelova et al. 1991a-c; Chiwakata et al. 1991; Kanchev et al. 1995; Middendorff et al. 1993). SP (Fig. 5.1b) is a member of the tachykinin family which comprises several vasoactive and smooth muscle cell contracting peptides. Both, Sertoli cells and Leydig cells express the preprotachykinin A gene (Chiwakata et al. 1991; Debeljuk et al. 2003). The most important tachykinins in mammals are SP, neurokinin A, neuropeptide K, neuropeptide γ and neurokinin B (see Debeljuk et al. 2003, for a review). The tachykinin receptors neurokinin 1 and neurokinin 2 have also been described in the testis.

SP was found in Leydig cells of human, hamster, guinea pig and Syrian hamster; however, we were not able to prove SP immunoreactivity in rat Leydig cells, thus providing evidence for species-related differences in the expression of this peptide (Angelova et al. 1991c; Chiwakata et al. 1991). In addition, we found transcripts of the preprotachykinin A gene in human and mouse, but not in rat and boar testes (Chiwakata et al. 1991). In the latter study, messenger RNA (mRNA) for both SP and neurokinin A receptors was detected in the human testis, raising the possibility that SP may act in an autocrine manner on Leydig cell function. Furthermore, we found that SP inhibits the testosterone production in isolated hamster Leydig cells (Angelova et al. 1991a, b) and, interestingly, that SP acts partially by modulating the binding capacity of luteinizing hormone (LH) in Leydig cells (Kanchev et al. 1995). Moreover, we were able to establish that both prepubertal and adult

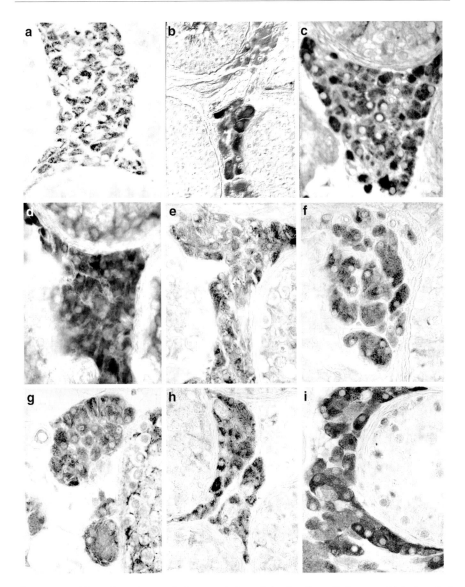

Fig. 5.1 Steroidogenic and neural characteristics of the Leydig cell. Immunohistochemical examinations revealed cytochrome P450 side chain cleavage enzyme (CytP450scc) (a), substance P (b), neuronal nitric oxide synthase (c), NADPH diaphorase (d), nerve growth factor β (e), p75[NGR] (f), TrkA (g), TrkC (h) and neurotrophin-3 (i) in adult human Leydig cells (× 350)

populations of Leydig cells in the hamster testis are SP-immunoreactive, suggesting, at least in this species, the absence of major alterations in the expression of SP during testis development (Angelova and Davidoff 1989; Angelova et al. 1991a, b). Remarkably, SP was found to exert different effects on the testosterone production by either prepubertal or adult Leydig cells (Angelova and Davidoff 1989; Angelova et al. 1991a, c). This fact may be explained by alterations in the structure of LHRs in these cells during development (Ge et al. 1996). Another testicular target cell for tachykinins seems to be the Sertoli cell. It has been reported that tachykinins modulate the secretory activity of rat Sertoli cells (Rao et al. 1995), supporting a paracrine role for SP and other tachykinins in the testis (see Debeljuk et al. 2003, for a review). Representing findings of separate importance (namely concerning the origin of Leydig cells), no differences in the activity for 3ß-hydroxysteroid dehydrogenase were detectable between intertubular and peritubular rat Leydig cells, since these cell populations were regarded at that time to derive from different cell lineages (Dupont et al. 1993).

As emphasized by Debeljuk et al. (2003), tachykinins may not only modulate the hypothalamo-pituitary axis, but have also direct influence on testicular cells by supporting intercell communications. Functionally, SP and other tachykinins have mainly an inhibitory effect on the testosterone secretion by Leydig cells. On the other hand, tachykinins possess the ability to stimulate the secretory activity of the Sertoli cells.

5.1.2.2
Neurotensin

Neurotensin, an endogenous tridecapeptide neurotransmitter, and its receptors were found in the central nervous system, the gastrointestinal tract and the cardiovascular system (Vincent et al. 1999; Tyler-McMahon et al. 2000) showing neurotransmitter, endocrine and paracrine properties. Neurotensin of the rat nervous system has an important impact on the release of acetylcholine, γ-aminobutyric acid (GABA), glutamate and taurine from the prefrontal cortex (Petkova-Kirova et al. 2008). We were able to demonstrate neurotensin immunoreactivity of variable intensity within the cytoplasm of human Leydig cells.

5.1.2.3
Neuropeptide Y

Further studies presumed that NPY may also modulate testicular function (Kopp et al. 2008). Kanzaki et al. (1996) provided evidence for the expression of mRNA^{NPY} in cultured immature rat Leydig and Sertoli cells and for the existence of a paracrine system for regulation of the NPY gene in the testis. The levels of mRNA^{NPY} increase after treatment with LH, FSH, interleukin-1α, interleukin-1ß, forskolin (an activator of adenylyl cyclase), and phorbol 13-myristate 12-acetate (an activator of protein kinase C). In Leydig cells, factors released from Sertoli and germ cells are also involved in the regulation of NPY gene levels. These results are of particular interest because NOS is colocalized with NPY, TH and vasoactive intestinal (poly) peptide (VIP) in nerves supplying the human ureter (Smet et al. 1994; Mayerhofer 2007). In adult human Leydig cells, relatively low amounts of NPY, VIP and peptide histidine isoleucine were detectable, and it seems likely that the maximum of NPY expression is found in immature Leydig cells (Davidoff, unpublished).

5.1.3
γ-Aminobutyric acid

The inhibitory neurotransmitter GABA, its synthesizing enzyme glutamate decarboxylase as well as GABA-A receptors were found not only in the central nervous system (in the developing brain, GABA regulates cell migration, differentiation and proliferation) but also in peripheral endocrine organs such as the developing and adult rat testes and in TM3 Leydig cells (Geigerseder et al. 2003, 2004; Doepner et al. 2005; Mayerhofer 2007). In the testis, GABA stimulates Leydig cell proliferation. Apparently, the master transcription factor egr-1 is involved in these processes (Doepner et al. 2005).

The GABA transporter I (GAT 1) was detected in rat and mouse testes, and its abnormal expression in mice seems to severely affect reproduction processes (Hu et al. 2004).

5.1.4
The NO/cGMP System

Recently, the main components of the NO/cGMP system were established in human Leydig cells (Davidoff et al. 1995, 1996; Rosselli et al. 1998; Davidoff and Middendorff 2000; Middendorff et al. 1997a, b, 2000). NO is a radical produced by a family of enzymes termed "nitric oxide synthases" (NOSs). One inducible and two constitutive isoforms are expressed in different organs and tissues. The constitutive isoforms, NOS-1 and NOS-3, require Ca^2/CaM and may be regulated by other factors such as protein kinase A, protein kinase C and Ca^{2+}/CaM PK II. The inducible, or macrophage, form of NOS (NOS-2) is Ca^2-insensitive and is activated by immunological or infectious stimuli and experimentally by substances such as lipopolysaccharide, interferon-γ, interleukin-1α, and TNF-α. We found moderate to strong immunoreactivity for NOS-I (Fig. 5.1c, d) and moderate to low immunoreactivity for NOS-3 and NOS-2 (Davidoff et al. 1995, 1996), suggesting the possibility that Leydig cells are able to produce NO under different circumstances. This fact and the accumulation of the second messenger cGMP after treatment of isolated human Leydig cells with the NO donor sodium nitroprusside (Davidoff et al. 1996) suggest that Leydig cells contain an active sGC representing the intracytoplasmatic receptor for NO (Middendorff et al. 1997a, b, 2000). In addition, a testis-specific variant of NOS-1 (TnNOS) was revealed in human and mouse Leydig cells (Wang et al. 1997, 2002). It was shown that NO inhibits testosterone secretion in rat Leydig cells (Adams et al. 1992; Welch et al. 1995; Mondillo et al. 2008). This inhibition is probably due to histamine-induced NOS activation (Mondillo et al. 2008). A possible paracrine influence of NO, produced by macrophages, on Leydig cell steroidogenesis as suggested by Weissman et al. (2005) cannot be excluded, but a reciprocal paracrine talk between neighbouring Leydig cells, between Leydig cells and other testicular cells as well an autocrine regulation seems more probable (Davidoff et al. 1995). In ovarian granulosa-lutein cells, NO was also found to directly inhibit activity of aromatase, which is responsible for the conversion of androgens to oestrogens (Van Voorhis et al. 1994). In addition, we found that human Leydig cells showed immunoreactivity for molecules involved in the regulation of NOS-1 activity, e.g. the excitatory amino acids glutamate and aspartate as well as the Ca^2-binding proteins CaM and Ca^{2+}/CaM PK II. In contrast to Sertoli cells, in which NOS-3 immunoreactivity was most intensive, NOS-1 clearly predominated in Leydig cells (see above). Recent findings suggest that some human cells can express the inducible NOS-2 gene constitutively (Park et al. 1996). It should be noted that NO mediates the action of numerous hormones (LH, LHRH, vasopressin, growth hormone) and neurotransmitters (SP, calcitonin gene related peptide, acetylcholine, noradrenaline, 5-HT, etc.) (Slusher et al.1994; Davidoff et al. 1995; Davidoff and Middendorff 2000, for a review). NO may also have cytotoxic properties if it is released in larger amounts and in combination with superoxide anions (Dawson 1995). The resulting molecule, peroxynitrite, is a highly toxic molecule that may account for apoptosis and degeneration of Leydig, Sertoli and germ cells. However, both Leydig and Sertoli cells exhibit immunoreactivity for superoxide dismutase (our unpublished data), suggesting that they are able to eliminate superoxide anions. Thus, a toxic effect of NO on these cells may be expected only at higher NO concentrations (Kukucka and Misra 1993, for guinea pig Leydig cells).

The lack of expression of NOS in rat Leydig cells seems to be characteristic for rats only, because in testes of other species (e.g. mice, Asian catfish, pig; Giannessi et al. 1998; Ruffoli et al. 2001; Davidoff and Middendorff 2000; Ambrosino et al. 2003; Nee Pathak and Lal 2008) and especially in man a functionally active endogenous NO/cGMP system was revealed (Davidoff et al. 1995, 1997a; Davidoff and Middendorff 2000). Different from the human testis (Davidoff et al. 1993), a large number of macrophages were found in rat (Hutson et al. 1990; Raburn et al. 1991; Nes et al. 2000; Lukyanenko et al. 2001). Moreover, Jorens et al. (1995) showed that in human macrophages the expression of NOS-2, in contrast to expression in other species, requires specific conditions, and limited quantities of NO appear to be generated via the L-arginine pendent effector pathway. The pattern of NOS and NADPH diaphorase (NADPH-d) staining in the mouse testis resembles the human, but not the rat one (Burnett 1995; Lissbrant et al. 1997). In accordance, Weissman et al. (2005) could not establish the expression of any form of NOS in rat Leydig cells (see also Burnett 1995), and Lissbrant et al. (1997) did not find any NADPH-d enzyme activity in rat Leydig cells, whereas in mouse Leydig cells both enzymes were found to be expressed (Davidoff et al. 1995; Davidoff and Middendorff 2000). However, in mouse MA-10 and TM3 Leydig cell lines an active sGC was missing, explaining the lack of NO effects in these Leydig cell lines (Davidoff et al. 1995, 1997a). In contrast, isolated human Leydig cells showed a dose-dependent increase of sGC-mediated cGMP production after incubation of cells with the NO donor sodium nitroprusside.

In our first publication dealing with testicular NO we discussed the endothelial localization of NOS and its functional significance (Davidoff et al. 1995). Lissbrant et al. (1997), however, established that NO only plays a limited role in the regulation of testicular blood flow under basal conditions (see Middendorff et al. 1997b). But NADPH-d activity increased after human chorionic gonadotropin (hCG) treatment, suggesting that NO was of importance for increasing the blood flow under these conditions (Lissbrant et al. 1997).

In summary, Leydig-cell-produced NO may (1) regulate the steroidogenic activity in an intracrine way (Del Punta et al. 1996), (2) modulate the action of neuropeptides, hormones, growth factors and cytokines in an autocrine way, (3) synchronize the functional activity of neighbouring Leydig cells in a paracrine way, (4) modulate the contractile activity of smooth muscle cells and vascular pericytes and regulate the blood flow rate and permeability of the vessels and (5) influence the contraction state of peritubular myofibroblasts, thereby contributing to the peristaltic activity of seminiferous tubules (NO produced by ectopic Leydig cells, which are found among myofibroblasts and smooth muscle cells in the tunica albuginea, may exert the same action and may be involved in the rhythmic contraction waves of the testicular capsule) (Davidoff et al. 1995). In addition, the NO signalling pathway participates in the control of testicular steroidogenesis during stress (Kostic et al. 1999). Moreover, in male rats, testosterone may activate NOS-1 in neurons of the medial preoptic area, resulting in an increase of local dopamine release, finally affecting their copulatory activity (Du and Hull 1999; Sato et al. 2005). Furthermore, there are important data showing that the mitotic activity of adult neural stem cells is negatively regulated by NO (Packer et al. 2003).

In contrast to the rat, human Leydig cells do not express hemoxygenase-2, which is responsible for the production of an additional cellular messenger, namely carbon monoxide, also leading to elevation of intracellular cGMP levels by activation of sGC (Davidoff et al. 1996; Ewing and Maines 1995). Therefore, it seems likely that carbon monoxide is not effective in the regulation of human Leydig cell function.

5.1.5
Neurotrophins and Their Receptors

Recent studies provide evidence that Leydig cells of the mammalian and human testes are involved in synthesis and release of a large number of biologically active substances that are typical for nerve cells and neuroendocrine cells (Davidoff et al. 1993, 1996; Middendorff et al. 1993; Russo et al. 1994; Seidl et al. 1996; Davidoff et al. 2001; Müller et al. 1999, 2006b). Neurotrophic factors are well-known extracellular signalling molecules in the central and peripheral nervous system that regulate neuron development, survival and maturation of neuronal phenotypes. In the rat testis, NGF protein and mRNA levels do not correlate with the innervations by NGF-sensitive nerve fibres, suggesting specific local functions for NGF within the male reproductive organ (Olson et al. 1987; Ayer-Lelievre et al. 1988). Several neurotrophins were found in adult and developing rat and mouse testes (Müller et al. 2006b). Using reverse transcription PCR (RT-PCR), western blot, immunohistochemical and functional analyses, Müller et al. (2006b) established expression and localization of the main neurotrophic factors and their receptors in human adult and differentiating Leydig cells and partially identified their functional role in morphogenesis and spermatogenesis. Immunoreactivity (with different staining intensity) for NGF, NT-3, NT-4 and BDNF as well as for $p75^{NTR}$, TrkA, TrkB and TrkC was observed mainly in the Leydig cells (Figs. 5.1e-i, 5.3a).

Previous studies suggested that TGF-β plays a key role in the regulation of neuron survival and death, and potentiates the neurotrophic activity of several neurotrophic factors. One of these factors is GDNF, which together with neurturin, persephin and artemin belongs to a class of proteins that is structurally related to the TGF-ß family (Lin et al. 1993; Baloh et al. 1998). It could be established that adult and differentiating human (15-34 weeks of gestation) and rat (5-90 postnatal days) Leydig cells express GDNF and its receptors GFRα-1 and GFRα-2. This study provides evidence for a functional implication of GDNF and its receptors within Leydig cells during their morphogenesis and further differentiation (Davidoff et al. 2001).

Neurotrophin signalling plays a role in the dynamic maintenance and differentiation of central nervous system endothelia (Kim et al. 2004), and $p75^{NTR}$ mediates neurotrophin-induced apoptosis of vascular smooth muscle cells (Wang et al. 2000). However, neurotrophins (as shown by local delivery of BDNF) can also promote revascularization in skeletal muscles by local recruitment of TrkB+ endothelial cells or by mobilization of TrkB+-expressing bone marrow haematopoietic progenitors (Kermani et al. 2005).

5.1.6
Catecholamines

The results concerning the existence of catecholamines in the Leydig cells of the human testis are controversial. The first information on the expression of catecholamine-synthesizing enzymes: TH (converting tyrosine into L-dopa), AADC (converting L-dopa into dopamine), DBH (converting dopamine into noradrenaline) and PNMT (converting the noradrenaline into adrenaline) in the Leydig cells of the human testis was reported by Davidoff et al. (1993, 1996) and Middendorff et al. (1993). In contrast, Mayerhofer et al. (1996, 1999) described a network of elongated neuronlike cells in prepubertal rhesus monkey (Frungieri et al. 2000) and in adult human testis (Mayerhofer et al. 1999). According to Mayerhofer (1996, 2007), Leydig cells of rodents do not produce catecholamines, but internalize them from peripheral autonomic nerves through the extracellular matrix. However, recent immunohistochemical studies by Romeo et al. (2004) provided evidence for TH and DBH expression in adult and infant Leydig cells. In a detailed study, Davidoff et al. (2005) provided strong evidence for the expression in human prenatal and adult Leydig cells of TH, AADC, DBH and PNMT, using RT-PCR analyses, in situ hybridization, western blot analyses and immunohostochemical amplification techniques as well as control sections from human substantia nigra and small peripheral nerves (Fig. 5.2a-f). It is important to emphasize that not all testes which were examined were found to express the main catecholamine-synthesizing enzymes simultaneously. This is in agreement with results published for other cell types. The results obtained by Davidoff et al.(2005) show that with regard to TH expression the Leydig cells show close similarity to catecholaminergic nerve cells. No adrenergic small neurons, as described by Mayerhofer et al. (1999), Frungieri et al. (2000) and Mayerhofer (2007), could be found in the prenatal and postnatal human testes. In this respect, it is possible

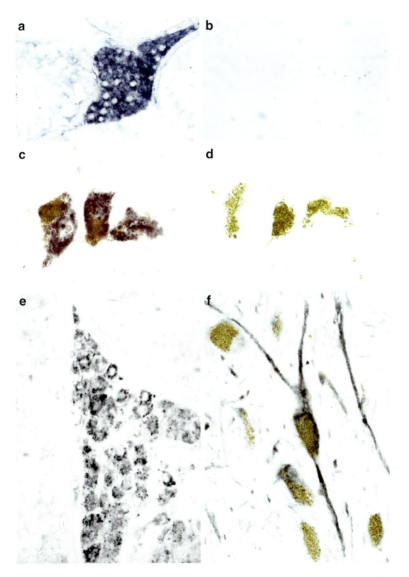

Fig. 5.2 Catecholamines in human Leydig cells. Gene expression of tyrosine hydroxylase (TH) in Leydig cells is demonstrated by in situ hybridization with an antisense probe (a). Sections treated with a sense probe were used to prove reaction specificity (b). To serve as a positive control, human mesencephalic substantia nigra was examined under the same experimental conditions. TH messenger RNA is detectable by blue-violet reaction products (c). The yellow-brownish staining on control sections, treated with sense probes, visualized the endogenous pigment of the nerve cells (d). Demonstration by immunohistochemistry of TH in Leydig cells of the human testis (e) and in the human substantia nigra, where the endogenous pigment appears yellow (f) (a, b ×160; c, d ×600; e ×350; f ×500)

that these authors (Mayerhofer et al. 1999; Frungieri et al. 2000; Mayerhofer 2007) considered the so-called compartmentalizing cells (Co-cells) of the testicular interstitium (Holstein and Davidoff 1997) as small neuronlike cells. These Co-cells phenotypically resemble glial cells of the nervous system and in analogy with neural glia they may be able to take up TH (and other neurotransmitters) released by neighbouring nerve fibres or Leydig cells (Davidoff et al. 2005).

5.2
Hormones

In human and rat Leydig cells, expression of thyrotropin-releasing hormone (TRH) and a partially inhibitory effect of TRH on LH/hCG-induced testosterone secretion were established (Feng et al. 1992; Montagne et al. 1996, Wilber et al. 1996). Moreover, in situ hybridization studies showed that within the testis, TRH receptor mRNA was exclusively detected in Leydig cells (Zhang et al. 1995). Thus, TRH represents an autocrine regulator of Leydig cells comparable to other hypothalamic neurohormones (GnRH, GHRH, proopiomelanocortin and CRH) (Fig. 5.3b).

After administration of triiodothyronine (T3) to prepubertal rats in order to induce hyperthyroidism, the number of interstitial mesenchymal cells was lower compared with the number in age-matched controls. Hypothyroidism inhibits Leydig cells regeneration, and hyperthyroidism results in accelerated differentiation of mesenchymal cells into Leydig cells following ethane dimethanesulphonate treatment (Ariyaratne et al. 2000b, c). Mendis-Handagama and Ariyaratne (2008) established that in prepubertal rats differentiation of adult Leydig cells is stimulated by thyroid hormone and inhibited by anti-Müllerian hormone from immature Sertoli cells. Thyroid hormone stimulation of adult Leydig cell differentiation, however, is not mediated by inhibition of anti-Müllerian hormone production. Teerds et al. (2007) observed that spindle-shaped stem Leydig cells undergo proliferation and differentiation under the influence of the thyroid hormone T3 and growth factors such as leukaemia inhibitory factor, stem cell factor, PDGF-A and EGF/TGF-α. Recently, the thyroid hormone receptors c-erbAα and c-erbAβ were found in regenerating rat Leydig cells after ethane dimethanesulphonate treatment by immunohistochemical methods, providing evidence for a role of T3 in Leydig cell

Fig. 5.3 (continued) peptide (c), glial fibrillary acidic protein (d), cyclic 2,3-nucleotide 3′-phosphodiesterase (e) and neural cell adhesion molecule (f). Arrows in e point to compartmentalizing cell processes. g, h Staining of Leydig cells by anti-CytP450scc. Note that the appearance (shape) of the Leydig cells is influenced by the direction of the sections. However, the basic form of the Leydig cells in rat testis at postnatal day 60 is bipolar (resembling the form of the pericytes, their ancestors), and processes of different length arise from both poles of their large oval cell bodies (g, arrows). Most of the processes are in direct contact with blood vessel walls or run parallel to the microvascular surface (h, arrows). At places where blood vessels are cross-sectioned (h, asterisks), adjacent Leydig cells show a round shape, and the processes cannot be recognized. (a ×350; b, c ×390; d ×450; e ×280; f ×370; g, h ×380)

Catecholamines

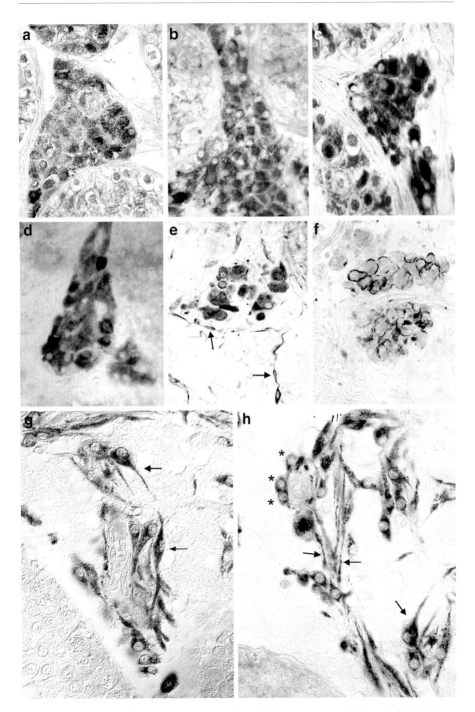

Fig. 5.3 Visualization of various antigens in the adult human testis (a-f) and of CytP450scc in rat testis at postnatal day 60 (g, h). Immunohistochemical approaches revealed brain-derived neurotrophic factor (a), growth-hormone-releasing hormone (b), C-type natriuretic

differentiation (Koeva et al. 2008b). A similar ontogeny pattern was proposed for the human fetal brain during the first trimester of its development (Iskaros et al. 2000). This finding is in agreement with an important role of thyroid hormones for brain development. The α TH receptor (TRα) is expressed in nestin-positive progenitor cells of the brain subventricular zone, providing evidence for a critical role of liganded TRα for neurogenesis in the adult mammalian brain (Lemkine et al. 2005). Moreover, hypothyroidism reduces proliferation of neural stem cells and limits their migration. Thyroid hormones also promote cell differentiation of human neuronal precursors (Benvenuti et al. 2008).

5.2.1
Melatonin

A new autocrine or paracrine regulator of Leydig cell function seems to be the neurohormone melatonin, an indole derivative (N-acetyl-5-methoxytryptamine) secreted by the pineal gland (Frungieri et al. 2005). Melatonin is synthesized from 5-HT. Melatonin-binding sites in the rat testis as well as an inhibitory effect of melatonin on gonadotropin-stimulated androgen synthesis have been established (Tijmes et al. 1996; Frungieri et al. 1999). Both 5-HT and TPH were localized to Leydig cells of the human (Davidoff et al. 1993) and golden hamster (Frungieri et al. 1999, 2002) testes. Additionally, structural changes in the testis were described after melatonin treatment of immature rats and mice (Ng and Ooi 1990; Olivares et al. 1989). Melatonin-binding sites were detected on rat Leydig cells (Vera et al. 1993), and the enzymes necessary for the local production of melatonin were detected in rat testis (Tijmes et al. 1996). Moreover, it was suggested that melatonin suppresses cyclic AMP (cAMP)-stimulated and non-cAMP-stimulated testosterone production in rat Leydig cells by reducing cAMP production or in part by inhibiting 17,20-desmolase activity (Valenti et al. 1995). However, prolonged exposure to melatonin results in sensitization of LH-dependent adenylyl cyclase activity. In this context, we were able to demonstrate moderate immunoreactivity for melatonin within the cytoplasm of the human Leydig cells.

5.3
Natriuretic Peptides

There is evidence that natriuretic peptides may influence testicular function via specific guanylyl cyclase A and (to a lesser extent) guanylyl cyclase B receptors (Schumacher et al. 1993; Tinajero et al. 1993a, b; Khurana and Pandey 1993; Mukhopadhyay et al. 1986; Pandey et al. 1984; Pandey 1994). Middendorff et al. (1996) detected mRNA for CNP, one member of the natriuretic peptide family, in human Leydig cells (Fig. 5.3c) and found that these cells also express transcripts of the corresponding receptor, the membrane-bound guanylyl cyclase B which generates the messenger cGMP, suggesting an autocrine/paracrine function of CNP in the human testis (Middendorff et al. 1997c, 2000a). In addition, we established moderate immunoreactivity for ANP and BNP in human Leydig cells, using particularly well characterized antisera against these peptides. In this respect, there is also evidence for the expression of ANP in Leydig cells of the rat, where it stimulates testosterone production in a time- and dose-dependent manner (El-Gehani et al. 2001; Pereira et al. 2008; see also Middendorff et al. 2000a, b; Müller et al. 2006a).

5.4
Neurofilament and Other Proteins

A characteristic component of neurons is the existence of typical neurofilament proteins which are components of the cellular cytoskeleton. Cytoskeletal proteins that were found in Leydig cells are microtubules, actin filaments and intermediate filaments of the vimentin type (Russell et al. 1981; Bilinska 1989; Schulze 1984). Davidoff et al. (1999) provided the first evidence that Leydig cells of the human testis express all necessary proteins required for the assembly of neurofilaments. By means of RT-PCR, western blot analyses and immunohistochemistry, these authors showed the existence of transcripts encoding for the neurofilament triplet proteins in isolated Leydig cells, and localized NF-H, NF-M and NF-L to the cytoplasm of Leydig cells in tissue sections (Fig. 7.4f). In addition, neurofilament proteins were also described in Sertoli cells of seminiferous tubules.

Another intermediate filament protein is nestin. Nestin was predominantly found in developing and regenerating rat and human Leydig cells (see below; Davidoff et al. 2004; Lobo et al. 2004). The demonstration of nestin expression within Leydig cells allowed Davidoff et al. (2004) to identify pericytes and vascular smooth muscle cells of the testis microvasculature as the stem/progenitor cells of Leydig cells. Nestin is predominantly expressed in activated stem/progenitor cells of various organs, and is especially found in the central and peripheral nervous system.

In addition to neurotrophins and neurofilament proteins, Leydig cells also express further characteristic proteins. One of them is presenilin-1. The presenilin gene is expressed in human brain, heart, liver, spleen, kidney and highest in testis (Suzuki et al. 1996). Presenilin-1 is expressed in neural progenitor cells of the hippocampus of adult mice (Wen et al. 2002, 2005). Presenilin-1 is also abundantly expressed during Leydig cell development (Yamaguchi et al. 2000). In addition, amyloid precursor protein gene promoter constructs are preferentially expressed in the central nervous system and testis of transgenic mice (Fox et al. 1997). In the nervous system, both presenilin-1 and amyloid precursor protein mark the early onset of the Alzheimer's disease. These results, once more, confirm the close relationship between neural structures and Leydig cells.

5.5
Astrocyte and Oligodendrocyte Marker Molecules

Another interesting fact is the occurrence of glial cell marker substances in Leydig cells of different species. The first evidence that Leydig cells of the Syrian hamster are immunopositive for the astrocyte marker GFAP was reported by Maunoury et al. (1991). GFAP belongs to the group of intermediate filaments found in cells of neural origin (astrocytes) as well as in numerous cell types of non-neural tissues. GFAP is expressed in steroidogenic cells of the adrenal cortex and in hamster Leydig cells (Maunoury et al. 1991). In a number of other species, including rat and human, these authors did not find any immunoreactivity for GFAP, suggesting species-dependent differences in the expression of this glial marker.

Two years later, Holash et al. (1993) found GFAP, glutamine synthetase, and S-100 protein immunoreactivity in rat Leydig cells located in the vicinity of testicular microvessels. Holash et al. (1993) proposed that the closeness of Leydig cells to the microvasculature supports the blood-testis barrier. This is comparable to the importance of astrocytes for the blood-brain barrier within the central nervous system. Davidoff et al. (1997b, 2002) performed a detailed study to establish whether other glial-cell-related substances are expressed by the testicular Leydig cells. Using immunohistochemistry and western blot techniques on material from adult (51-86 years of age) and developing (15th-36th weeks of gestation) human testes, Davidoff et al. (2002) established GFAP (astrocyte marker) (Fig. 5.3d), GalC (expressed by oligodendrocytes and Schwann cells), CNPase (expressed by oligodendrocytes and Schwann cells) (Fig. 5.3e), A2B5 (represents GT3 and other c-series gangliosides expressed by oligodendrocytes, type II astrocyte progenitor cells, some neurons and neuroendocrine cells) and O4 antigen (sulphated glycolipids and seminolipids expressed by progenitor O4$^+$ GalC$^-$ glial cells that differentiate further towards GalC$^+$ oligodendrocytes) immunoreactivity in human Leydig cells, thus providing evidence that Leydig cells of the human testis, in addition to their endocrine, neuronal and neuroendocrine features, possess qualities of both astrocytes and oligodendrocytes of the nervous system. The results obtained supported the view that fetal and adult Leydig cells share a common origin.

There are no data on the possible functional significance of these marker substances. A possible role of GFAP for the intracellular transport of cholesterol in steroidogenesis (Maunoury et al. 1991) and of cytoskeletal filaments in intracellular signalling (Forgacs 1995) was suggested.

5.6
The Renin-Angiotensin System

Despite some controversy concerning the renin-angiotensin system of the human testis (Mukhopadhyay et al. 1995), it seems likely that human Leydig cells possess prorenin, renin (Deschepper et al. 1986), angiotensin I, angiotensin-converting enzyme (Pandey et al. 1984), angiotensin II and angiotensin receptor I immunoreactivity, providing evidence for the existence of an additional autocrine/paracrine regulatory system. Interestingly, patients pretreated with anti-androgenic drugs showed reduced angiotensin II immunoreactivity (Ergün et al. 1999).

Recently, an intrinsic renin-angiotensin system of the brain was suggested, which regulates numerous physiological processes, such as blood pressure control (Grobe et al. 2008; Ito et al. 2008). In the brain, neurons, expressing angiotensin II, affect other nerve cells through the activation of angiotensin receptors and/or via generation of NO and reactive oxygen molecules (Carlson and Wyss 2008).

The Leydig cells also express NCAM that was found in the human testis on the surface of the Leydig cells (Mayerhofer et al. 1992, 1996; Davidoff et al. 1993) especially in zones where two cells are in contact with each other (Fig. 5.3f).

Two other important factors for Leydig cell development as well as brain development and function are VEGF and PDGF.

5.7
VEGFs and Their Receptors

The VEGF and its receptors VEGFR-1 (Flt-1) and VEGFR-2 (Flk-1; human counterpart, KDR) are important regulators of and play an essential role for physiological vasculo- and angiogenesis (Ferrara et al. 2003; Yamada and Takakura 2006; Wakui et al. (2006). In the normal human testis, Ergün et al. (1997) found VEGF in Leydig and Sertoli cells, but not in testicular vasculature. VEGFR-1 (Flt-1) was found in Leydig cells, Sertoli cells and in perivascular cells, and also in a population of endothelial cells, whereas VEGFR-2 (KDR) was detectable in endothelial cells, perivascular cells, Leydig cells and Sertoli cells. The authors concluded that VEGF plays an essential role as a paracrine mitogenic and angiogenic factor in modulation of capillarization, maintenance of the function of microvasculature and control of permeability of testicular capillaries. In the testis, ovary, adrenal glands and placenta, two novel, highly related VEGF homologues, Bv8 and endocrine-gland-derived VEGF (EG-VEGF), were revealed. In the testis, their receptors are present in endothelial cells, where they promote angiogenesis and mobilization of peripheral blood cells (LeCouter et al. 2003, 2004). EG-VEGF, Bv8 and their receptors have also been described in the central nervous system and a certain relevance for angiogenesis was presumed (Ferrara et al. 2004). In the testis, the high proliferation rate of endothelial cells may be affected by these VEGF homologues, suggesting continuous remodelling of testis microvasculature (Collin and Bergh 1996). In addition, Beckman et al. (2006) demonstrated that VEGF is expressed in capillary pericytes of the developing corpus luteum, and others have shown that FGF2 and angiopoietins are present in the corpus luteum. VEGF and FGF2 target endothelial cells to initiate angiogenesis and to stimulate NO production. Conversely, NO may increase VEGF expression by vascular smooth muscle cells and pericytes. NO caused a dose-dependent increase in VEGF, FGF2, ANGPT2 (angiopoietin 2) and GUCY1B3 (guanlyate cyclase 1, Soluble, beta 3) mRNA expression in ovine luteal pericytes. Expression of mRNA for ANGPT1 (angiopoietin1) in luteal pericytes was not affected by NO treatment. These data provide further evidence for a role of luteal pericytes and NO in the expression of angiogenic factors, and of potential interactions of pericytes with endothelial cells by NO production (see also Kobayashi et al. 2006, showing that hepatocyte growth factor mediates angiopoietin-induced smooth muscle cell recruitment).

VEGF is an important factor of neurogenesis (Fabel et al. 2003). In addition, VEGF represents a haemoattractant for FGF2-stimulated neural progenitors (Zhang et al. 2003; Fabel et al. 2003) and promotes their proliferation via the cell-cycle-related gene E2F (Zhu et al. 2003).

Recently, it has been demonstrated that pericytes represent an important source of VEGF and may migrate in a defined relationship to endothelial cells, which guide the sprouting processes (Ozerdem and Stallcup 2003). Endothelial cells produce PDGF-B, which in turn attracts PDGFR-B+ perivascular cells to the walls of growing blood vessels (Lindahl et al. 1997b). Perivascular cells, such as smooth muscle cells and pericytes, wrap around the vessels, providing structural support and regulating endothelial cell function.

5.8
PDGFs and Their Receptors

PDGFs are members of the PDGF-VEGF family of growth factors (see Mariani et al. 2002, for a review). Four PDGF forms are known: PDGF-A, PDGF-B, PDGF-C and PDGF-D. The active PDGF forms are either homodimers or heterodimers. Two types of PDGF cell surface receptor tyrosine kinases (PDGFR-α and PDGFR-ß) have been established in different tissues. PDGF receptors dimerize, and have different binding capacity. The B receptor only binds PDGF-BB; the A/B receptor binds AA, BB and AB dimers (Hart et al. 1988).

The PDGF variants have numerous functional effects on target cells: proliferation, migration, contraction, extracellular matrix production, differentiation and survival (Mariani et al. 2002).

In the testis, members of the PDGF family and their receptors (PDGF-A, PDGF-B, PDGFR-α and PDGFR-ß) were found during prenatal and postnatal life (Gnessi et al. 1992, 1995). During testis development, PDGFs and their receptors are produced by Sertoli cells and peritubular myofibroblasts (Puglianiello et al. 2004). In the adult rat, however, only Leydig cells express PDGF-A, PDGF-B, PDGFR-α and PDGFR-ß. PDGF-B and PDGFR-ß mutant mice lack vascular smooth muscle cells, pericytes and glomerular mesangial cells (Hellström et al. 1999). Recently, Fecteau et al. (2008) described that PDGF-A was first detectable at postnatal day 10 and localized to Leydig cell progenitors at a peritubular position, but not to mesenchymal or any other spindle-shaped cells in rat interstitium. The authors suggested that expression of PDGF-A in Leydig progenitor cells may be associated with proliferation and migration of these cells away from the peritubular region during Leydig cell differentiation.

The reduction of PDGF-A could account for the reduced Leydig cell number in androgen receptor knockout mice and Sertoli-cell-specific androgen receptor knockout mice (Tan et al. 2005). Analysis of expression patterns and characterization of the gonad phenotype in PDGFR-α (−/−) embryos identified PDGFR-α as a critical mediator of signalling in the early testis at multiple steps of testis development. PDGFR-α XY (−/−) gonads displayed disruptions in the organization of the vasculature and in the partitioning of interstitial and testis cord compartments. Closer examination revealed severe reductions in characteristic XY proliferation, mesonephric cell migration and fetal Leydig cell differentiation, identifying PDGF signalling through the α receptor as an important event downstream of Sry in testis organogenesis and Leydig cell differentiation (Brennan et al. 2003). Moreover, PDGF-A (−/−) mice show gross impairment of adult Leydig cell development (Brennan et al. 2003).

Using Wnt1-Cre and Sox10-Cre mice crossed to Rosa26^{Yfp} reporter mice, Foster et al. (2008) revealed neural-crest-derived mesenchymal cells in the adult murine thymus and found that neural-crest-derived cells infiltrate the thymus before day 13.5 of embryonic development and differentiate into cells with characteristics of smooth muscle cells associated with large vessels, and pericytes associated with capillaries. In the adult organ (3 months of age), these neural-crest-derived perivascular cells continue to be associated with the vasculature, providing structural support to the blood and possibly regulating endothelial cell function. The neural-crest-derived cells in the thymus express PDGF receptors that are characteristic of mesenchymal cells. Both PDGFR-α and PDGFR-ß are preferentially expressed by cells of mesenchymal nature, including pericytes. PDGFR-ß is required for recruitment of pericytes to the wall of blood vessels.

Turnbull and Rivier (1997) provided evidence for the existence of a direct neural-testicular connection. They proposed that the inhibitory effects of centrally injected (intracerebroventrcular) interleukin-1β on Leydig cell testosterone production are not mediated by suppression of LH secretion or the result of increases in glucocorticoids. Instead, they suggested that loss of testicular responsiveness to LH is due to direct brain-to-gonad connections that bypass the pituitary (Turnbull and Rivier 1997).

Taken together, the information presented above shows unequivocally that Leydig cells are not only androgen-producing cells, but contain a large number of marker substances characteristic for neural and neuroendocrine cells. This fact strongly supports the concept of the neuroendocrine nature of both fetal and adult Leydig cells.

Chapter 6
Development of the Testis

Before the new aspects concerning the origin, morphology and functional features of the Leydig cells are focused upon, a brief survey of the origin and differentiation of the main structural components of the testis is presented.

6.1
The Testis Arises from the Urogenital Ridge and the Indifferent Gonad Rudiment

The mammalian gonad develops within the urogenital ridge as a thickening along the ventromedial cranial area of the mesonephros. In mice, this occurs at day 10.0–10.5 post coitus (dpc) (Byskov 1986; Brennan and Capel 2004; Kim and Capel 2006; Wilhelm et al. 2007; Tang et al. 2008). This thickening results from both the proliferation of the coelomic epithelium and the allocation of cells from the mesonephros (Yao and Capel 2002; Ross and Capel 2005; Cool et al. 2008). At the beginning, the structure of this gonad anlage is identical in XX and XY mice embryos, and either ovary or testis can develop from this bipotential primordium. For testis development, a member of the Sox (Sry-related high-mobility group box) family of transcription factors, SRY (sex-determining region of the Y chromosome; Sry in mice) is expressed as a primary trigger by the supporting cell lineage, the precursor cells to the Sertoli cell lineage (DiNapoli and Capel 2008). Between 11.5 and 12.5 dpc in mice, the following events were established in the XY gonad: increased proliferation of coelomic epithelial cells, migration of cells from the mesonephros, structural organization of the testis cords, appearance of a male-specific coelomic vessel and differentiation of the steroidogenic Leydig cells (Brennan and Capel 2004).

6.2
Primordial Germ Cells Migrate from the Epiblast into the Genital Ridges

In mice, primordial germ cells (PGCs) can be identified at 6.0–6.5 dpc in the epiblast close to the extraembryonic ectoderm (Wilhelm et al. 2007) and at the base of the allantois and the forming hindgut around 7.0–7.5 dpc (Chiquoine 1954; Ginsburg et al. 1990). The PGCs divide, migrate through the gut mesentery and the aorta-gonad–mesonephros region and enter the developing gonad (urogenital ridges) between 9.5 and 11.5 dpc (DiNapoli et al. 2006; corresponding to 5–10-week-old human embryos, He et al. 2007). Until this stage of development (about 10.5 dpc), mouse XX and XY gonads and germ cells behave in an identical manner with respect to their formation, proliferation and migration. The gonocyte number at 11.5 dpc is about 3,000 (Tam and Snow 1981), and gonocytes continue to proliferate until 13.5 dpc, when they enter meiosis in ovaries or mitotic arrest in testes (McLaren 2000, 2003; Adams and McLaren 2002). Remarkably, recent results provide evidence that the germ cell lineage passes through a series of differentiation steps (epigenetic modifications) before giving rise to oogonia and spermatogonia. It is important to note that reprogramming of the PGCs begins prior to their migration into the genital ridge (at embryonic day 8.0–8.5 and prolongs during migration, embryonic day 9.5, and still after they have colonized the genital ridge, embryonic day 11.5, 12.5) (Yamazaki et al. 2003; Durcova-Hills et al. 2006; Shovlin et al. 2008).

In the human fetal testes, Bendsen et al. (2003) calculated the number of germ cells and somatic cells during the first weeks (weeks 6–9 after conception) after sex differentiation. The number of germ cells increased from about 3,000 in week 6 to about 30,000 in week 9. The ratio of germ cells to Sertoli cells was about 1:11 and the ratio of germ cells to somatic cells was about 1:44 throughout this period. At week 7, the total number of somatic cells was about 600,000 and increased to 1,750,000 in week 9. The number of Sertoli cells at week 7 was about 150,000 and increased to about 450,000 in week 9.

6.3
The Sertoli Cells Emerge from Migrating Cells of the Coelomic Epithelium and Contribute to the Formation of the Testicular Cords

In addition to the PGCs, somatic cells also differentiate in the developing gonads in a sex-specific manner (XY or XX). In the male (XY) testis, Sertoli cell progenitors (the "supporting cell lineage") originate from multipotent cells in the coelomic epithelium between embryonic days 10.5 and 11.5 under the influence of Sry, formerly termed the "cell-autonomous testis-determining factor" (TDF) of the Y chromosome (Karl and Capel 1998; Wilhelm et al. 2005, 2007). These cells proliferate in the coelomic epithelium between embryonic days 11.3 and 11.5 (Schmahl et al. 2000). Following delamination, they start to express Sry messenger RNA, which is necessary for the differentiation of the progenitors into differentiated Sertoli cells (Bitgood et al. 1996; Wilhelm et al. 2007). The male-specific somatic Sertoli cells are important for testis development (McLaren 1991, 1998; Brennan and Cappel 2004). While Sry expression in mice gonads is initiated at 10.5 dpc, the male pathway and the structural discrimination from the female gonad appear at 12.0 dpc (Park and Jameson 2005; Di Napoli et al. 2006).

The process of the sex-specific development is accompanied by upregulation within the Sertoli cells of additional factors (Wilhelm et al. 2007), such as the Sry-like Sox9 (Wright et al. 1995; Bishop et al. 2000; Vidal et al. 2001; Koopman 2005; Wilson et al. 2006), desert hedgehog (Dhh) (Bitgood et al. 1996; Yao et al. 2002), platelet-derived growth factor receptor α (PDGFR-α) (Brennan et al. 2003), anti-Müllerian hormone (AMH) (Behringer et al. 1994), fibroblast growth factor 9 (FGF9) (Colvin et al. 2001; Kim et al. 2006), steroidogenic factor 1 (SF1), a nuclear receptor encoded by Nr5α1 (Sf1) (Park et al. 2007; Sekido and Lovell-Badge 2008), the retinoic acid degrading enzyme CYP26B1 (a cytochrome P450 enzyme that prevents oogenesis in males by retarding meiosis in vivo; Bowles et al. 2006), Wnt4 and possibly RSPO1 (see Brennan and Capel 2004; Park and Jameison 2005; DiNapoli and Capel 2008, for reviews).

As mentioned above, the gonad primordium is morphologically indistinguishable in males and females (indifferent, bipotential) from 10.0 through 11.5 dpc (Wilhelm et al. 2007). At 12.0 dpc, Sertoli and germ cells coalesce and become surrounded by a layer of peritubular myofibroblast cells, thereby contributing to the formation of the testicular cords (Buehr et al. 1993; Merchnat-Larios et al. 1993; Martineau et al. 1997; Capel et al. 1999; Brennan et al. 2002, 2003; Jeanes et al. 2005). The differentiation of the testicular cords occurs rapidly. In the rat, for example, it takes approximately 24 h (Byskov 1986). At this stage, the testis comprises two main compartments: the testicular cords and the intertubular space (the interstitium) between them (Brennan and Capel 2004; Jeanes et al. 2005). Proliferation of germ and somatic precursor cells in XY individuals promotes enlargement of the testis at about 13.5 dpc (Park and Jameson 2005).

6.4
Migrating Mesonephric Cells Contribute to the Generation of Other Somatic Cells in the Male Gonad

The fate of other cell types in the gonad depends on cellular activities of supporting progenitors. Cells, producing either female or male steroid hormones, differentiate after specification of the supporting cell lineages. In the male gonad, a population of steroid-hormone-producing somatic cells, the Leydig cells, develops. These cells are distributed within the interstitium among the testis cords (the future seminiferous tubules) and around the blood vessels of the testis.

At 11.5–16.5 dpc, the Sox9 gene is upregulated, leading to a massive migration of mesonephric cells finally destined to become peritubular myofibroblasts, vascular endothelial cells and myoepithelial (perivascular) cells (Buehr et al. 1993; Martineau et al. 1997; Tilmann and Capel 1999; Brennan et al. 2002; Brennan and Cappel 2004; Coveney et al. 2008). The vascular endothelial cells become organized in a testis-specific coelomic vessel (Yao et al. 2006; Coveney et al. 2008; Cool et al. 2008), and subsequently the interstitial Leydig cells arise (Brennan and Capel 2004; Tang et al. 2008). Crucial factors necessary for the early development of the Leydig cells are Dhh and Pdgfr-α as well as the homeobox gene aristaless-related (ARX) (Brennan et al. 2003; Brennan and Capel 2004). The results obtained by Colvin et al. (2001) showed that exogenous Fgf9 induces mesonephric cell migration into embryonic day 11.5 XX gonads, suggesting that Fgf9 in the early testis could act also as a chemotactic factor for mesonephric cells. Mesonephric cells that migrate into the testis proliferate (Martineau et al. 1997), suggesting that the same signals induce both migration and proliferation (Colvin et al. 2001).

Chapter 7
Development of the Neuroendocrine Leydig Cells

7.1 Two Main Leydig Cell Types Differentiate During Testis Development: The Fetal-Type and the Adult-Type Leydig Cells

The question concerning the origin of the Leydig cells has been addressed for a long time and leads to controversial results. Principally, two main types of Leydig cells have been recognized during development of animal and human testes, namely the fetal-type Leydig cells that differentiate during prenatal development and the adult-type Leydig cells which arise in the postnatal period of testis development (Roosen-Runge and Anderson 1959; Lording and de Kretser 1972; Christensen 1975; Hardy et al. 1989; Kuopio et al. 1989a-c; Benton et al. 1995; Pelliniemi et al. 1996; Ariyaratne and Mendis-Handagama 2000; Ariyaratne et al. 2000a; Haider 2004; Yao and Barsoum 2007; Ge and Hardy 2007; Ge et al. 2006; Teerds and Rijntje 2007). There is substantial evidence that Leydig cells represent a heterogeneous cell population not only during development but even in adulthood (Davidoff et al. 1996). The different populations of Leydig cells exhibit diversity in size, organelle composition, physicochemical properties and metabolic activity (Christensen 1965; Schulze 1984; Purvis et al. 1979).

The adult Leydig cells comprise two populations, namely immature-adult Leydig cells and mature-adult Leydig cells (Prince 2001; Ge et al. 2006; Ge and Hardy 2007; Teerds and Rijntjes 2007; Teerds et al. 2007). In the postnatal human and rat testis, an additional phenotype was recognized - the so-called fetal-type Leydig cells thought to represent a continuation of the embryonal fetal Leydig cells until adulthood (Kerr and Knell 1988; Pelliniemi et al. 1996).

Most of the authors assume that the two main (fetal and adult) types of Leydig cells are separate cell lineages of different origin (Kerr and Knell 1988; Brennan and Capel 2004; Haider 2004; Ge et al. 2006; O'Shaughnessy et al. 2008a, b). Recently, this was proposed on the basis of studies on gene expression during development (Ge et al. 2005; Dong et al. 2007; Zhang et al. 2008). However, there is also considerable evidence for a great similarity regarding the generation and differentiation of fetal and adult Leydig cells (Benton et al. 1995; Teerds and Rijntjes 2007; Teerds et al. 2007; Ge et al. 2005, 2006; Dong et al. 2007; Tang et al. 2008).

Following the discovery of the Leydig cells (more than 150 years ago), nearly all somatic cellular components of the testis were presumed to be the ancestors of the Leydig cells. In addition, most of the publications regarding the origin of the Leydig cells point to a multifocal origin (Russell et al. 1995; Russell 1996; Yao and Barsoum 2007; Ge and Hardy 2007). The postulated origin includes mesenchymal-like stem cells (Huhtaniemi and Pelliniemi 1992; Hardy et al. 1989; Benton et al. 1995; Ge et al. 1996; Teerds 1996; Ariyaratne et al. 2000a; Mendis-Handagama and Ariyaratne, 2001; Haider 2004), fibroblast-like cells (Mancini et al. 1963), peritubular myoid/fibroblast cells (Russell et al. 1995; Haider et al. 1995; Chemes 1996), macrophages (Clegg and Macmillan 1965) as well as (based exclusively on morphologic observations) connective tissue cells that include lymphatic endothelial cells, perivascular fibroblast-like cells and pericytes (Jackson et al. 1986; Kerr et al. 1987b; Russell et al. 1995; Jégou and Pineau 1995). At present, the hypothesis prevails that the Leydig cell progenitors represent spindle-shaped mesenchymal-like cells of the testicular interstitium with predominantly peritubular location (Benton et al. 1995; Ariyaratne et al. 2000a; Mendis-Handagama and Ariyaratne 2001; Yao and Barsoum 2007; Ge and Hardy 2007; Teerds et al. 2007). However, the latter location was recently questioned by O'Shaughnessy et al. (2008b).

Recent investigations addressing the regenerative capacity of testicular Leydig cells identified vascular smooth muscle cells and pericytes of the testis microvasculature as progenitors of all postnatal Leydig cell phenotypes. Remarkably, these cells are distinguished by expression of the intermediate filament protein nestin (a marker for neural and other stem/progenitor cells) (Davidoff et al. 2004). After depleting the existing Leydig cell population of adult rats by a single injection of ethane dimethanesulphonate (EDS), pericytes (and smooth muscle cells) of the testis microvasculature initially proliferate (self-renew), detach from the vessel wall (migrate) and transdifferentiate into new/young (blast, progenitor) Leydig cells which after additional division steps develop into adult Leydig cells (Benton et al. 1995; Ge and Hardy 2007; Teerds and Rijntjes 2007; Teerds et al. 2007).

In the following, we discuss in detail the origin of the adult population of Leydig cells after depletion by EDS treatment (Teerds 1996; Teerds et al. 1999, 2007; Teerds and Rijntjes 2007) as well as the Leydig cell generation during postnatal development (Benton et al. 1995; Ge and Hardy 2007; Teerds et al. 2007). In the next chapter we shall discuss the origin and development of the fetal Leydig cells.

7.2
Origin and Differentiation of the Adult Neuroendocrine Leydig Cells

It is now well accepted that both fetal-type and adult-type Leydig cells originate from stem cells (Benton et al. 1995; Ge et al. 2006; Tang et al. 2008). Two main sources are proposed: mesenchymal stem cells and vascular mural cells of the testis (pericytes and smooth muscle cells), but their exact nature remains unresolved. This is especially true for the mesenchymal stem cells of the testis because mesenchyme represents a mixture of cells which may originate from all three embryonal germinal layers (ectoderm, mesoderm and endoderm) (Chemes 1996).

The postnatal development of the Leydig cell lineage comprises different types of differentiating cells: stem Leydig cells, precursor Leydig cells, progenitor Leydig cells and adult Leydig cells. The latter can be subdivided into immature-adult and mature-adult Leydig cell stages (Hardy et al. 1989; Shan et al. 1997; Ge and Hardy 2007; Teerds and Rijntjes 2007; Teerds et al. 2007; Zhang et al. 2008).

7.3
Definition and Classification of the Stem Cells

Taking into account certain controversies in the literature concerning the definition of the stem cells, a short recapitulation of the classification of stem cells will be presented (Weissman 2000; Weissman et al. 2001; Rosenthal 2003; Rao 2004a, b; Biswas and Hutchins 2007; Morrison and Spreadling 2008; Zhang et al. 2008; Ratajczak et al. 2008).

Stem cells are single cells that are clonal precursors of both more stem cells of the same type, as well as a defined set of differentiated progeny (Weissman et al. 2001). Stem cells can be roughly classified in three main categories according to the time of their isolation during ontogenesis: embryonic, fetal and adult (Marcus and Woodbury 2008).

As is well known, fertilization of an ovum initiates the development of an embryo from a zygote. The zygote undergoes constant divisions or cleavage and sequentially reaches a stage termed "morula" (containing four to 32 cells). The morula grows and migrates further within the uterine tube and arrives in the uterine cavity, where it builds a vesicular formation termed "blastocyst", or "blastula", a structure comprising a central cavity surrounded by a double cell wall (the trophoblast) and an excentrically situated accumulation of cells within the fluid-filled cavity. This cell accumulation is termed the "inner cell mass", or "embryoblast". The inner cell mass further becomes reorganized into two cell layers: one layer adjacent to the trophoblast (termed "epiblast") and one adjacent to the central cavity of the blastocyst (termed "hypoblast"). The epiblast gives rise to the amnion prior to gastrulation and also differentiates towards the three primary fetal germ layers from which the whole embryo arises: ectoderm, mesoderm and endoderm. Gradually these epiblast precursors mature into organ- and tissue-specific somatic stem cells. The hypoblast provides the extraembryonic tissues, embryonic endoderm and the extraembryonic mesoderm which surrounds the amniotic membrane and the yolk sac and it also participates in the generation of the placenta, which is a product of the trophectoderm.

7.3.1
Embryonic Stem Cells

Two types of embryonic stem cells were recognized, namely early and late (blastocyst) embryonic stem cells.

The early embryonic stem cells comprise the cells of the zygote and the morula up to the 16-cell stage (Suwiska et al. 2008). These cells are totipotent. "Totipotent" means that a single cell from these structures is able to produce a new embryo, including the extraembryonic tissues (the trophoblast, including the placenta).

The late embryonic stem cells comprise the cells from the inner cell mass of the blastocyst. These cells are pluripotent. "Pluripotent" means that these cells are capable of giving rise to any cell type of the body except for the extraembryonic tissues (the trophoblast, including the placenta). Recently, Ilancheran et al. (2007) revealed that human stem cells derived from human fetal membranes (amniotic epiblast cells) represent a reservoir of stem cells with characteristics of human embryonic stem cells.

7.3.2
Fetal Stem Cells

During fetal development the so-called fetal stem cells represent descendants of the late embryonic stem cells. These cells are pluripotent and able to differentiate into all cells and tissues before birth of an individual. An example for fetal stem cells is the umbilical cord blood and matrix with its haematopoietic and mesenchymal stem cells. In the fetal nervous system, fetal neural stem cells were found to have radial morphology, known as radial glia (Okano 2002a, b). The radial glia produces neurons and glial cells and guides the newly produced cells to their final destination, thereby contributing to histogenesis of the organ. Fetal stem cells also reside within extraembryonic (extracorporeal) tissues: amniotic fluid, amniotic membrane, Wharton's jelly of the umbilical cord and the placenta (Ilancheran et al. 2007; Marcus and Woodbury 2008, for a review).

7.3.3
Adult Stem Cells

Adult stem cells are organ-specific inconspicuous cells which are multipotent and responsible for the growth, maintenance, physiological replenishment and regeneration of the organs after degenerative diseases and injury. A characteristic feature of these cells is their plasticity, which means the capability to transdifferentiate into other cell types of the organism depending on local environmental factors (Vescovi et al. 2002; Rosenthal 2003). Another feature of adult stem cells is their ability to differentiate not only into terminally differentiated cells, but also to dedifferentiate (Jiang et al. 2003, 2004; Bailey et al. 2006; Kanatsu-Shinohara et al. 2004). Adult stem cells were described in the gonads (germline stem cells and mesenchymal testicular stem cells), in the skin (epithelial stem cells), in the central nervous system (CNS), in the skeletal muscle, in intestine, liver, heart, pancreas, retina, peripheral nervous system and in the bone marrow (haematopoietic stem cells and mesenchymal/stromal stem cells). Mesenchymal/stromal stem cells appear disseminated throughout the adult organism (da Silva Meirelles et al. 2006, 2008; Nardi 2005).

Adult stem cells can be dormant (quiescent, silencing or low proliferating) within restricted tissue regions termed "stem cell niches". Such cells can be activated under certain conditions involving the generation of an intermediate, fast-proliferating cell population called the "transit amplifying compartment" (Vescovi et al. 2002; Doetsch 2003a; Morrison and Spradling 2008).

7.4
Postnatal Development of the Neuroendocrine Leydig Cells in Rat and Mouse Testis

During both normal postnatal development and regeneration after EDS application, different types of Leydig cells were detectable in the rat testis: fetal Leydig cells, stem/progenitor Leydig cells, precursor Leydig cells, fetal-type and spindle-shaped progenitor Leydig cells and adult Leydig cells, the latter differentiating into immature-adult and mature-adult Leydig cells (Benton et al. 1995; Hardy et al. 1989; Ariyaratne et al. 2000a, 2003; Davidoff et al. 2004; Teerds and Rijntje 2007; Teerds et al. 2007; Ge and Hardy 2007). A possible reciprocal inhibitory relationship between the number of fetal-type and differentiating adult Leydig cells was suggested (Ariyaratne et al. 2000b; Ariyaratne and Mendis-Handagama 2000).

7.4.1
New Data Concerning the Stem/Progenitor Cells of the Adult Leydig Cell Lineage

In the current literature, the origin of the Leydig cells is still a matter of debate (Hardy et al. 1989; Teerds 1996; Benton et al. 1995; Teerds et al. 1999, 2007; Ariyaratne and Mendis-Handagama 2000; Ariyaratne et al. 2000 a, b; Mendis-Handagama and Ariyaratne 2001; Haider 2004, 2007; Ge et al. 2006; Yao and Barsoum 2007; Dong et al. 2007). Moreover, owing to difficulties in the clear-cut identification of the Leydig cell progenitors (Myers and Abney 1991), the results concerning the origin and early differentiation of the Leydig cells are often contradictory (Myers and Abney 1991; Gaytan et al. 1992; Hardy et al. 1989; Benton et al. 1995; Teerds et al. 1999, 2007; Ariyaratne et al. 2000a, b; Zhang et al. 2008).

At present, a consensus has arisen that the stem Leydig cells are mesenchymal cells located within the testicular interstitium (Habert et al. 2001). In this regard, it is important to note remarkable neuroendocrine properties (neuronal and glial) of Leydig cells. This was revealed in rat, mouse, hamster and human testis, and a possible neuroectodermal/neural crest origin of these cells was proposed (Schulze et al. 1987a; Angelova and Davidoff 1989; Angelova et al. 1991c; Chiwakata et al. 1991; Davidoff et al. 1993, 1996, 2001; Middendorff et al. 1993; Benton et al. 1995).

In support, Mayerhofer et al. (1992, 1996) and Mayerhofer (2007) showed by in situ hybridization, western blots and immunohistochemistry the expression of the neural cell adhesion molecule (NCAM) as well as of some other neural marker molecules in testicular Leydig cells of adult rats, mice and hamsters.

7.4.1.1
The EDS Model for Adult Leydig Cell Regeneration Represents an Excellent Tool To Study the Postnatal Development of the Testicular Leydig Cells

Animal experiments leading to regeneration of a depleted Leydig cell population after single intraperitoneal EDS administration in the rat contributed essentially to the understanding of the normal postnatal development of adult Leydig cells (Kerr et al. 1985, 1986, 1987a, b; Teerds 1966; Teerds and Rijntjes 2007; Teerds et al. 2007). There is broad evidence that the regeneration process after EDS administration recapitulates the postnatal ontogenesis of the Leydig cells in the rat (Teerds 1996; Yan et al. 2000; Davidoff et al. 2004; Teerds and Rijntjes 2007; Teerds et al. 2007; Koeva et al. 2008a, b). Of particular advantage, in EDS-treated rats, distinct phases of Leydig cell regeneration are clearly distinguishable, whereas during postnatal development these phases partially overlap and can be less clearly distinguished (Davidoff et al. 2004; Teerds and Rijntje 2007). Thus, the possibility to destroy all existing Leydig cells in the adult rat testes by EDS helps to distinguish individual developmental stages, to identify and localize Leydig stem/progenitor cells and to follow up the fate of regenerating Leydig cells (Kerr et al. 1985, 1986, 1987a, b; Molenaar et al. 1985; Benton et al. 1995; Teerds 1996; Teerds et al. 1999, 2007; Teerds and Rijntje 2007).

EDS, a diester of methane sulphonate, is a bifunctional alkylating substance. A single intraperitoneal application of EDS at a dose of 75 mg kg^{-1} weight destroys the existing population of Leydig cells and leads to a decline in blood testosterone concentration (Jackson et al. 1986; Morris et al. 1986; Morris et al. 1997; Kerr et al. 1985, 1987a, b; Klinefelter et al. 1991; Teerds 1996; Teerds et al. 1999, 2007; Teerds and Rijntje 2007). Between 2 and 4 days after EDS injection, all testicular Leydig cells undergo apoptosis and are eliminated from the intertubular space by macrophages accumulated in their vicinity. During the following 3 weeks, Leydig cells regenerate, and a completely new population of these cells arises.

Fig. 7.1 (continued) at day 21 after EDS injection (**b**). Asterisks indicate microvessels, T seminiferous tubules. **c**–**f** Selected longitudinal sections of microvascular vessels showing the transition of precapillaries to capillaries. Demonstration of 5-bromo-2′-deoxyuridine incorporation in nuclei of a periendothelial vascular smooth muscle cell (*arrow*) and pericytes (*asterisks*) (**c**), nestin immunoreactivity in periendothelial vascular smooth muscle cells (*arrows*) and pericytes (*asterisks*) (**d**), high molecular weight melanoma-associated antigen (NG2) immunoreactivity in pericytes (*arrows*) of a capillary wall (**e**) and α-smooth muscle actin immunoreactivity in vascular smooth muscle cells and pericytes (*arrows*) of a microvessel (*asterisk*) (**f**) (**a** ×500; **b** ×700; **c** ×1,000; **d** ×800; **e** ×520; **f** ×650). (**a, c**–**f** Modified from Davidoff et al. 2004)

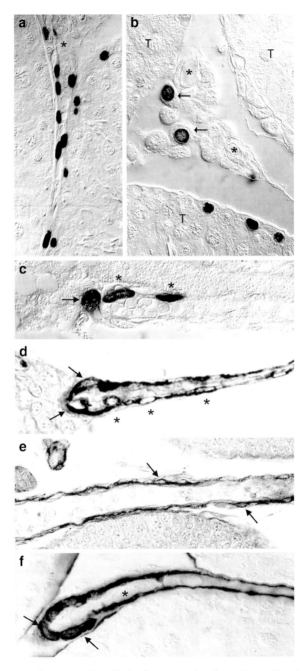

Fig. 7.1 Generation of new Leydig cells in the rat testis after ethane dimethanesulphonate (EDS) administration. Proliferation of the Leydig cell stem cells (pericytes and smooth muscle cells) at day 2 (**a**) and of young differentiating Leydig cells (Leydig cell progenitors; arrows)

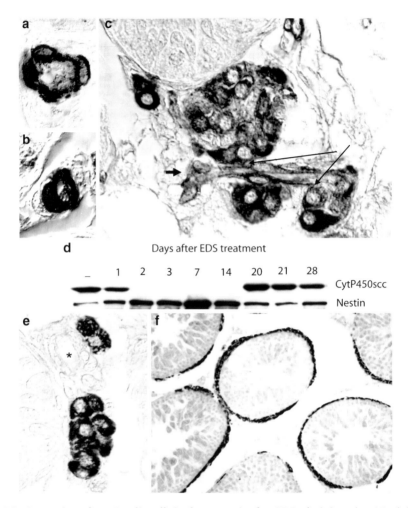

Fig. 7.2 Generation of new Leydig cells in the rat testis after EDS administration. Nestinimmunoreactive pericytes begin to protrude from microvessel walls at day 14 after EDS injection (**a, b**) and migrate to form cell clusters (**c**) in the direct vicinity of the vessel (orientation indicated by a *thick arrow*). Nestin-positive cells that are still in contact with the capillary from which they derive are indicated (**c**, *thin arrows*). Immunoblot analyses demonstrate increased nestin expression during the period of Leydig cell depletion (indicated by the disappearance of cytochrome P450 cholesterol side chain cleavage enzyme, CytP450scc) (**d**). Visualization of fetal-type Leydig cell aggregates with strong CytP450scc immunoreactivity at day 14 after EDS administration (**e**, *asterisk* indicates a capillary). On day 21 after EDS treatment, a large number of young Leydig cells (Leydig cell progenitors) are detectable around seminiferous tubules (**f**). (**a** ×1,300; **b** ×880; **c** , **e** ×950; **f** ×550). (Data derived from Davidoff et al. 2004)

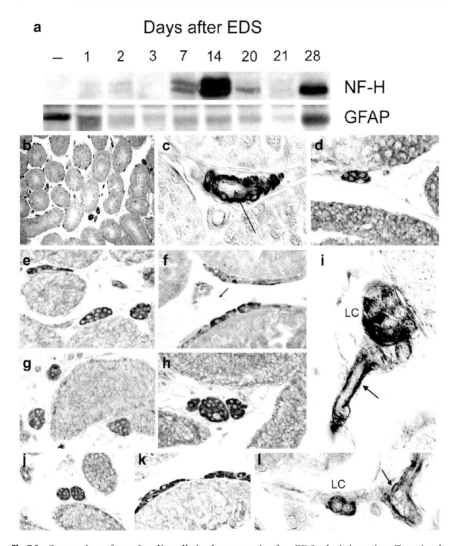

Fig. 7.3 Generation of new Leydig cells in the rat testis after EDS administration. Transiently elevated levels of NF-H and a reduced expression of glial fibrillary acidic protein (GFAP) in response to EDS-induced Leydig cell depletion are shown by immunoblotting (a) Newly formed Leydig cells as well as vascular smooth muscle cells and pericytes are immunoreactive for NF-H (b, c) GFAP (d) growth associated protein 43 (e) glial cell line derived neurotrophic factor (f) NeuroD (g), platelet-derived growth factor receptor ß (i) TrkA (j, k) and NG2 (l) at days 14 (b - e, i, j, l) or 21 (f, k) after EDS injection. Arrows mark unstained endothelial cells (c) and pericytes (j, l). LC Leydig cells(l). (b ×55; c ×350; d ×230; e ×200; f – h ×170; i ×630; j, k ×150; l ×380). (a – e Modified from Davidoff et al. 2004)

Four main phases of Leydig cell regeneration after EDS application have been reported (Benton et al. 1995; Ge et al. 2006; Zhang et al. 2008). In agreement with and supporting these results, Davidoff et al. (2004) elucidated the following distinct events:

1. Proliferation of stem/progenitor cells during the first week after EDS application with a peak at days 2 and 3 [established by immunohistochemical characterization of 5-bromo-2′-deoxyuridine (BrdU) incorporation] (Fig. 7.1a-c).
2. Transdifferentiation of the stem/progenitor cells into new Leydig cells (young or blast cells; similarly to young neurons or neuroblasts of the nervous system) at day 14 after EDS injection (Figs. 7.2a-c, 7.3). Some of these progenitor Leydig cells resemble the prenatal fetal Leydig cells. They are mostly situated within the intertubular space and were termed "fetal-type" Leydig cells (Fig. 7.2c, e). At the same time, only sporadically at intertubular and peritubular positions, spindle-shaped progenitor Leydig cells were also observed.
3. Around days 20-21 after EDS treatment, a large number of progenitor Leydig cells arise by transdifferentiation from stem/progenitor cells at peritubular positions, most frequently around tubules with damaged spermatogenesis (Fig. 7.2f). A small number of these cells contained BrdU in their nuclei, suggesting that at least some young (progenitor) Leydig cells start to divide rapidly following their emergence (Fig. 7.1b).
4. The young (progenitor, blast) Leydig cells differentiate further until the 60th day after EDS application into immature-adult and mature-adult Leydig cells (Ge and Hardy 2007; Teerds and Rijntje 2007).

7.4.1.2
Leydig Cells, After EDS Treatment, Originate from Microvascular Stem Cells After a Phase of Stem Cell Proliferation (Self-Renewal)

Substantial progress in understanding the Leydig cell development after EDS treatment was derived from a recent study (Davidoff et al. 2004), where the following experimental strategies were involved:

1. Labelling of dividing cells and the progenitor Leydig cells by means of BrdU incorporation
2. Immunohistochemical analyses of the Leydig-cell-specific protein cytochrome P450 cholesterol side chain cleavage enzyme (CytP450scc), the rate-limiting enzyme of steroidogenesis that is responsible for the conversion of cholesterol to pregnenolon to mark the cells of the Leydig cell lineage
3. Taking into account the neural properties of the Leydig cells, assessment of the expression of the neuronal stem cell marker nestin in rat Leydig stem/progenitor cells and in nestin-green fluorescent protein transgenic mice (Fig. 7.3c, d)
4. Examination by immunohistochemistry and western blot techniques of a number of neuronal and glial cell marker substances within the progenitor and adult Leydig cells
5. Performance of double immunohistochemical stainings to allow examination of transformation processes

7.4.1.3
Leydig Stem/Progenitor Cells Proliferate Mainly on Days 2 and 3 After EDS Treatment: Experiments with ^{3}H-Thymidine

It is well accepted that the mature-adult Leydig cells of the testis are postmitotic cells (Myers and Abney 1991; Benton et al. 1995). In addition, adult Leydig cells retain certain neuroendocrine qualities of their progenitors and resemble non-dividing adult nerve cells (Schulze et al. 1987a; Davidoff et al. 1993, 1996, 1997, 1999, 2001, 2002; Middendorff et al. 1993; Müller et al. 2006).

Previous studies in EDS-treated rats showed that spindle-shaped mesenchymal-like cells actively divide, doubling their number approximately every 7 days (Benton et al. 1995). During rat postnatal development (between days 14 and 28), mesenchymal-like cells also proliferate, but their total number decreases, suggesting a concomitant transformation into a new cell type. By day 14, a subset of these ^{3}H-thymidine labelled cells become progenitors committed to the Leydig cell lineage (Benton et al. 1995). Between days 14 and 28, during the first two phases of differentiation, about 50% of the adult quantity of Leydig cells are generated as progenitor cells. These cells transform between days 28 and 56 into adult-immature Leydig cells, which subsequently differentiate into adult Leydig cells. According to this investigation (Benton et al. 1995), a residual number of mesenchymal-like stem cells persist in adult animals. Peak values of ^{3}H-thymidine labelled Leydig cells and mitotic figures in Leydig cells were found at days 4, 21 and 22 after EDS administration by Teerds and Rijntje (2007). Yan et al. (2000) established three peaks of BrdU incorporation in the mesenchymal stem cells of EDS-treated rats after a single BrdU injection: the first peak at days 3 and 4 (when the mature Leydig cells were almost completely depleted), the second peak at day 10 (when serum testosterone had declined to undetectable levels and germ cells were extensively undergoing apoptosis) and the third peak at around day 20 (when testosterone levels had increased significantly in comparison with those on days 2-10).

7.4.1.4
Pericytes and Smooth Muscle Cells of the Testicular Microvasculature and Spermatogonia of Seminiferous Tubules Are the Only Cells in Rat Testis That Incorporate BrdU in Their Nuclear DNA Within 2 h After EDS Administration

To establish whether the stem-cell-like progenitor cells of the testis vasculature proliferate concomitant with enhanced nestin immunoreactivity (see later), Davidoff et al. (2004) injected BrdU intraperitoneally into rats at days 2, 3, 20 and 21 after EDS administration. Two hours after BrdU administration at days 2 and 3 following EDS injection, a strong labelling of numerous nuclei of pericytes and vascular smooth muscle cells of the intertubular and the peritubular segments of the testicular microvasculature was observed (Fig. 7.1a-c). After that, from day 14 onwards, the stem-cell-like progenitors transform into fetal-type and spindle-shaped adult Leydig cell progenitors. A second transdifferentiation phase was observed between days 20 and 21 leading to the appearance of a larger number of new (young, blast) progenitor Leydig cells. In contrast to the BrdU labelling during the first week after EDS treatment, at days 20 and 21 the number of labelled nuclei in the peritubular interstitium was lower, and most of the cells that resemble larger vascular smooth muscle cells or even differentiating young Leydig cells, located in the vicinity of the larger intertubular blood vessels, possessed BrdU-labelled nuclei (Fig. 7.1b). These results provided evidence that Leydig stem/progenitor cells proliferate mainly during the first 2-3 days after EDS treatment, and after reaching a defined number, their proliferation ability decreased. On day 21, only a minor number of proliferating stem/progenitor cells showed BrdU nuclear staining. In addition, at this time certain new progenitor Leydig cells with stained nuclei were detectable (Fig. 7.1b), suggesting a certain proliferation activity of these cells. The latter results are consistent with data obtained by histoautoradiography with ^{3}H-thymidine (Hardy et al. 1989; Teerds et al. 1999). A strong proliferation rate of pericytes, established by ^{3}H-thymidine incorporation in the rat testis after EDS administration, has been reported to coincide with two proliferation waves of interstitial mesenchymal cells (Teerds 1966). Ariyaratne and Mendis-Handagama (2000) reported also an increase of pericyte number until day 28 during rat testis development. However, these authors accepted only the mesenchymal cells as the Leydig cell progenitors.

7.4.1.5
The Time Period of Leydig Cell Depletion After EDS Treatment Is Characterized by Elevated Nestin Expression in the Stem/Progenitor Cells of Testicular Leydig Cells

Nestin represents an intermediate filament protein, showing close evolutionary relationship to neurofilament proteins (Dahlstrand et al. 1992a, b; 1995). Nestin is well established as being expressed in stem/progenitor cells of the developing and adult CNS (Messam et al. 2000; Kuhn et al. 2001; Almazan et al. 2001; Liu et al. 2002), CNS tumours (Dahlstrand et al. 1992b) as well as in the peripheral nervous system, skeletal muscle and some other organs (Sejersen and Lendahl 1993; Sjöberg et al. 1994; Frisén et al. 1995; Hunziker and Stein 2000; Mujtaba et al. 1998; Sommer 2001; Zulewski et al. 2001; Lechner et al. 2002). Nestin is expressed in proliferating stem cells and during their transition into differentiating lineage descendants (see later).

Immunohistochemically, nestin was seen exclusively in pericytes and smooth muscle cells of the testicular blood vessels as well as (with rapidly decreasing intensity) in the cytoplasm of the young (blast, progenitor) Leydig cells (Figs. 7.1d, 7.2a-c). The microvascular stem/progenitor cells showed also high molecular weight melanoma-associated antigen (NG2) and α-smooth muscle actin (αSMA) immunoreactivity (Fig. 7.1e, f). Increases in nestin-immunoreactive smooth muscle cells and pericytes occurred between days 2 and 3, as well as around day 14 and days 20-21 following EDS administration (Davidoff et al. 2004). This time course of elevated nestin immunoreactivity coincides with published results on ^{3}H-thymidine and BrdU incorporation into the nuclei of rat mesenchymal-like interstitial cells following EDS administration (Hardy et al. 1989; Myers and Abney 1991; Gaytan et al. 1992; Teerds 1996; Teerds et al. 1999; Davidoff et al. 2004). Fourteen days after EDS administration, nestin-positive cells protrude from the vessel walls (Fig. 7.2a, b) and accumulate in their vicinity in the form of clusters (nodules) representing the fetal-type Leydig cells that are described in the following section by visualization of CytP450scc immunoreactivity (Fig. 7.2e, f). On appropriate sections, the Leydig cell clusters were observed to be still in contact with the blood vessel walls from which they originate, and numerous fetal-type Leydig cells in the nodules showed nestin immunoreactivity (Fig. 7.2c). The newly formed progenitor Leydig cells rapidly lose their nestin immunoreactivity. Thus, a number of the regenerating Leydig cells in these clusters were nestin-negative and other cells showed immunoreactivity of decreasing staining intensity. On day 14 after EDS treatment, single nestin-positive spindle-shaped cells in peritubular positions were detectable. A second wave of accumulation of nestin-immunoreactive smooth muscle cells and pericytes in the walls of the testicular microvasculature was observed at days 20 and 21 after EDS administration.

Fetal-type Leydig cells expressing exclusively nestin, exclusively CytP450scc or both proteins could be established by double staining (Fig. 7.4e). In addition, Leydig cells of certain clusters also showed traces of αSMA immunoreactivity. These results provided substantial evidence that the progenitor Leydig cells originate by transdifferentiation from the microvascular pericytes and smooth muscle cells (Davidoff et al. 2004).

Comparative immunoblot analyses, performed with soluble fractions of testis homogenates, revealed low levels of nestin in normal (untreated) 3-month-old rats but relatively large amounts of nestin in EDS-treated rats, with the highest levels at day 7 after EDS administration (Davidoff et al 2004). Nestin levels for all time periods examined (days 1-47 after EDS administration) were much higher than in untreated rats, indicating that EDS exposure rapidly induces a massive nestin expression and that this effect is long-lasting. Thus, Leydig cell disappearance clearly coincides with elevation, and Leydig cell reappearance with diminution of nestin expression (Fig. 7.2d).

7.4.1.6
Nestin Is Widely Expressed in Activated and Proliferating Stem Cells

Both neural stem cells and stem cell progenitors of Leydig cells temporarily express nestin. However, nestin is not expressed exclusively by these cells. Nestin expression was also found in non-neural cells such as bone marrow stem cells, pancreatic stem cells, liver stem cells, skeletal muscle stem cells and hair follicle sheath progenitor cells (Vaittinen et al. 1999; Zulewski et al. 2001; Li et al. 2003). A common feature of nestin-positive cells is that they show different degrees of activation, which includes proliferation, rapid changes of their phenotype and migratory activity (Zimmerman et al. 1994; Dahlstrand ct al. 1995; Sahlgren et al. 2001; Vaittinen et al. 1999, 2001;

Almazan et al. 2001). In some organs, e.g. the skeletal musculature, nestin is associated with neural transmission or structures participating in neural transmission (Vaittinen et al. 2001).

7.4.1.7
Regenerating and Developing Young Leydig Cells Immediately Acquire a Steroidogenic and Neural Phenotype and Become Immunoreactive for Neuronal, Glial and Neuroendocrine Marker Substances

To define the time frame at which the new population of Leydig cells acquires steroidogenic and neural properties, the expression and localization of CytP450scc as well as of a number of biologically active substances that are characteristic for neural and neuroendocrine cells were analysed (Davidoff et al. 2004).

7.4.1.8
Immunohistochemical and Immunoblot Analyses of CytP450scc Expression After EDS Treatment

The only structures in the testis that displayed immunoreactivity for CytP450scc were the Leydig cells (Davidoff et al. 2004). CytP450scc completely disappeared 3 days after EDS treatment and began to reappear at the earliest 14 days after EDS injection. These cells were detected primarily as clusters of large, round and hypertrophic cells (resembling the fetal Leydig cells) located at the vicinity of intertubular vessels as well as in the form of single, peritubularly distributed spindle-shaped cells in the vicinity of peritubular capillaries. At this time, the total amount of Leydig cells was still very low, and an expression of CytP450scc was not yet detectable by immunoblotting (Fig. 7.1d).

On day 21 following EDS administration the number of CytP450scc-positive peritubular Leydig cell progenitors rapidly increased. Seminiferous tubules, in which the spermatogenesis was still impaired, were nearly entirely surrounded by a ring of two or more layers of young (blast, progenitor) Leydig cells (Fig. 7.2f). Leydig cell hypertrophy and/or hyperplasia was shown to occur in the vicinity of seminiferous tubules with impaired spermatogenesis, but not elsewhere in the testis (reviewed by Sharpe 1983, 1986). Between days 30 and 45 after EDS administration, and with improvement of spermatogenesis in seminiferous tubules, the number of peritubular progenitor Leydig cells decreased, and Leydig cell clusters were found predominantly within intertubular columns of testicular connective tissue, surrounding the larger vessels of the testicular microvasculature. This distribution pattern closely resembles the distribution pattern of Leydig cells of the normal mature rat testis.

The destruction and regeneration of Leydig cells following EDS treatment was confirmed by immunoblot analyses, demonstrating the absence of the 52-kDa CytP450scc protein at days 7 and 14 and its reappearance at days 20 and 28 after EDS injection (Davidoff et al. 2004) (Fig. 7.2d).

7.4.1.9
Leydig Cells Arise by Transdifferentiation from Microvascular Pericytes/Smooth Muscle Cells

In newly produced Leydig cells, the expression of nestin and alpha smooth muscle actin is lost rapidly and is replaced by gene products responsible for steroidogenic, neuronal and glial characteristics (Davidoff et al. 2004), indicating a fast transdifferentiation process. In accordance, only a few cells still showing expression of nestin (marker of the progenitors) and already expression of CytP450scc (steroidogenic marker of the Leydig cells) became detectable by double immunostaining (Davidoff et al. 2004). This fast transdifferentiation obviously hindered the recognition of the relationship between the pericytes and the Leydig cells in previous investigations (Teerds et al. 2007; Ge et al. 2006). It now appears that the development of Leydig cells comprises a sequential processes in which during prenatal development, Leydig stem/progenitor cells transdifferentiate into fetal Leydig cells, whereas during postnatal testis development, the Leydig stem/progenitor cells transdifferentiate into new (newborn, young, blast, progenitor) Leydig cells. After several mitotic divisions, beginning around postnatal day 56, they differentiate into the adult Leydig cell population (Ge et al. 2006; Ge and Hardy 2007; Dong et al. 2007; Teerds and Rijntje 2007; Teerds et al. 2007).

It has to be noted that recent publications characterized the stem cells of Leydig cells as mesenchymal-like cells situated within the peritubular and perivascular interstitium of the testis (Ge et al. 2005, 2006, 2007; Ge and Hardy 2007; Teerds et al. 2007). These so-called mesenchymal-like stem cells and/or side population stem cells (Yazawa et al. 2006; Lo et al. 2004) described morphologically and biochemically in these reports may represent early descendants of the Leydig stem/progenitor cells rather than a separate stem cell lineage. In addition, experimental manipulations such as isolation from testis tissue, sorting and culturing under different conditions to induce differentiation (Abney and Zhai 1998; Lo et al. 2004; Ge et al. 2006; Ge and Hardy 2007; Dong et al. 2007) can substantially affect their inherent properties and fate. For example, culturing under certain conditions can elicit reprogramming of otherwise committed cells (Blanpain et al. 2004; Li et al. 2004). As reported by Park et al. (2008), human and murine fibroblasts can be reprogrammed directly to pluripotency yielding the so-called induced pluripotent stem cells. The Leydig stem/progenitor cells do not express substances that are characteristic for differentiated Leydig cells (Davidoff et al. 2004; Ge et al. 2005; Ge and Hardy 2007). However, when pericytes in the testis leave their microvascular niche, they lose the protective function of the vascular stem cell niche and become activated. As a result, the pericytes divide, cease the expression of a number of genes and switch rapidly towards the expression of genes characteristic for the Leydig cell precursors, the immature (young, blast) Leydig cells and the adult Leydig cells (Ge et al. 2005, 2006; Ge and Hardy 2007; Teerds et al. 2007; Dong et al. 2007). In addition, during tissue preparations for isolation of the Leydig stem/progenitor cells, single free pericytes together with (more abundant) circulating and migrating mesoangioblasts, bone marrow cells, local stem cells and/or haematopoietic stem cells may accrue. Thus, such cell preparations may represent a complex mixture of interstitial mesenchymal stem cells. Both adult and fetal tissues contain mesenchymal stem/stromal cells ("multipotential mesenchymal stromal cells", Horwitz et al. 2005). These cells were found in bone marrow (Bianco et al. 2001), dental pulp (Gronthos et al. 2002; Shi and Gronthos 2003), the paravascular region of the periodontal ligament (Chen et al. 2006), adipose tissue (Zannettino et al. 2007a), myocardium (Martens et al. 2006), peripheral blood (Doyle et al. 2006; Rochefort et al. 2006), skeletal muscle (Tamaki et al. 2005; Péault et al. 2007; Dellavalle et al. 2007), skin (Pablos et al. 1999; Slack 2000; Toma et al. 2001; Li et al. 2003, 2004; Blanpain and Fuchs 2006), brain (Jiang et al. 2002), liver (Niki et al. 1999; Mancino et al. 2007; Yovchev et al. 2008), pancreas (Zulewski et al. 2001; Hunziker and Stein 2000), placenta (Battula et al. 2007), lung (Sabatini et al. 2005), umbilical cord (Ortiz-Gonzalez et al. 2004; Sarugaser et al. 2005; Marcus and Woodbury 2008), fetal and adult testis (Ge et al. 2006) as well as the connective tissue (Lo et al. 2004; Covas et al. 2008) and vascular wall and perivascular tissue of the testis and other organs (Cossu and Bianco 2003; Zengin et al. 2006; Chen et al. 2006; Ergün et al. 2007; Covas et al. 2008). Thus, these cells are ubiquitously distributed in the body (Reyes et al. 2001, 2002, 2003). When multipotent mesenchymal stem/stromal cells are placed in culture media, they become activated, start to proliferate and differentiate depending on the epigenetic factors present in these media (Covas et al. 2008). In an appropriate culture medium, these cells may differentiate towards progenitors or precursors of the Leydig cells (Ge et al. 2006; Teerds et al. 2007; Lo et al. 2004). Whether such cells represent the stem/progenitors for the Leydig cells during testis development in situ or after experimental ablation of the adult Leydig cell population with EDS remains questionable. Note that proliferating mesenchymal stem/stromal cells from the bone marrow express CD271 (neurotrophin receptor p75^{NTR}) (Bühring et al. 2007). The depletion of this receptor prevented differentiation of hepatic stellate cells, which were defined as hepatic pericytes (Pinzani et al. 1992), into myofibroblasts and abrogated the promotion of hepatocyte proliferation in a model of liver injury (Passino et al. 2007).

Considering that mesenchymal stem/stromal cells and pericytes are related cells located in the subendothelial and perivascular layers of the vasculature where they function as cell sources and for tissue maintenance (Covas et al. 2008), a characterization of Leydig cell stem cells as cells of mesenchymal origin was obvious. However, this disregards the fact that the mesenchyme represents embryonic connective tissue, comprising a mixture of cells originating from all three germinal layers, the ectoderm, mesoderm and endoderm (Chemes 1966). As shown (Davidoff et al. 2004), only the pericytes seem to be situated in a true vascular stem cell niche and are surrounded by a basal lamina. The basal lamina is regarded as an obligatory component of stem cell niches at least in the CNS, where it provides signals and molecules that are necessary for the maintenance of the stem cells within the niche (Mercier et al. 2002; Alvarez-Buylla and Lim 2004). The testicular microvascular pericytes proliferate after activation and show a progeny towards smooth muscle cells and Leydig cells, consistent with properties of stem cells. In EDS-treated rats, it became evident that the pericytes comprise resting (silencing) cells situated within the microvascular niches (Muffler et al. 2008). Following activation, they start to proliferate (self-renew), migrate out from the vascular niches and differentiate into smooth muscle cells, young (immature, blast) Leydig cell progenitors and mature Leydig cells. From a general point of view, pericytes in different organs differentiate towards a broad progeny (e.g. osteocytes, chondrocytes, adipocytes, smooth and striate muscle cells, neurons and glial cells) depending on local environmental factors, and they represent pluripotent stem cells with the capability, after transplantation, to give rise to various cell types characteristic for the host organ. In the testis, the fate of the pericytes appears restricted by their transdifferentiation into young (blast, immature) Leydig progenitor cells and smooth muscle cells of the vascular wall (Davidoff et al. 2004). No other cell type with mitotic activity in the testis (Russell et al. 1995; Teerds 1996) shows signs for such a transdifferentiation into Leydig cells.

7.4.1.10
Neuroendocrine (Neuronal and Glial) Marker Substances in Newly Appearing Leydig Cells

Very fast after their generation by transdifferentiation from pericytes/vascular smooth muscle cells, newly formed Leydig progenitor cells begin to express not only steroidogenic enzymes (CytP450scc) but also a large number of neuronal and glial cell antigens (Fig. 7.3a-l) such as neuroD, neuron-specific enolase, growth associated protein 43, microtubule-associated protein 2, synaptophysin, neurofilament protein 200 (NF-H), neuronal nuclei antigen, glial cell line derived neurotrophic factor (GDNF) and its receptor GRFα-2, platelet-derived growth factor B (PDGF-B) and its receptors PDGFR-ß and PDGFR-α. Furthermore, the cells become immunoreactive for the neurotrophic factor receptors TrkA, TrkB and TrkC and for the surface adhesion molecule NCAM. Glial-cell-specific antigens that are detectable include glial fibrillary acidic protein (GFAP), 2′,3′-cyclic nucleotide 3′-phosphodiesterase, A2B5 antigen and O4 antigen. In regenerating Leydig cells after EDS treatment as well as in Leydig cells during different periods of postnatal development, also immunoreactivity for vascular endothelial growth factor (VEGF), basic fibroblast growth factor (FGF2) and transforming growth factor β (TGF-ß) arises. Thus, immediately after their formation, newly produced Leydig cells acquire the neuroendocrine characteristics that are typical for mature Leydig cells of adult species, including man (Davidoff et al. 1993, 1996, 2002; Middendorff et al. 1993; Müller et al. 2006).

In conclusion, Leydig cells are generated by transdifferentiation of pericytes/vascular smooth muscle cells, representing a common stem-cell-like progenitor cell population. Newly formed Leydig cells acquire a steroidogenic as well as a neuroendocrine phenotype and rapidly lose nestin and αSMA immunoreactivity. The immediate decline of nestin and αSMA in the newly produced Leydig cells argues for the existence of highly effective cellular regulation mechanisms. Supported by

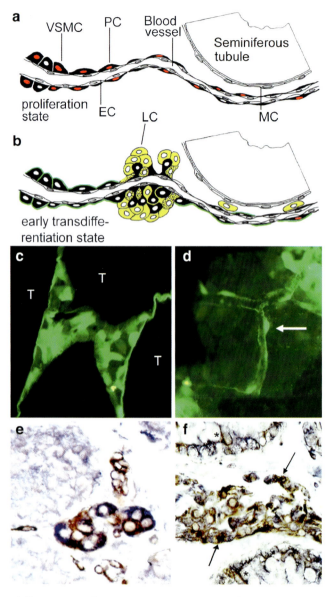

Fig. 7.4 Transdifferentiation of vascular progenitors into Leydig cells as discovered in therat/EDS model and investigations in mice and human. **a, b** The transdifferentiation process. Nestin-expressing (*black*) vascular smooth muscle cells (VSMC) and pericytes (PC) of testicular blood vessels, but not endothelial cells (EC) or peritubular myoid cells (MC), proliferate (indicated by *red-labelled nuclei*) during the first week after EDS-induced Leydig cell depletion (a). Around day 14 after EDS treatment, nestin-expressing vascular smooth muscle cells and pericytes, now transiently also expressing neurofilament protein 200 (NFH) (*green contour line*), begin to protrude from intertubular vessels and to form cell clusters (**b**). The cells first acquire steroidogenic properties (*yellow, black-dotted*) and

preliminary investigations, the ubiquitin/proteasome system probably contributes to this regulation. Thus, all Leydig cell phenotypes are characterized by both mesenchymal and neural (neuronal and glial) cell properties (Davidoff et al. 1996), indicative of neuroendocrine cells.

7.4.2
Young Leydig Cells Are Surrounded by Basement Membrane Fragments, Supporting Their Origin from Perivascular Pericytes

Typical pericytes are surrounded by a basement membrane, produced by both endothelial cells and the pericytes themselves (Sims 1991) and representing an important component of the pericyte vascular niche. Some previous reports showed the existence of basement membrane fragments on the surface of Leydig cells in fetal, newborn and postnatal rats (Kuopio and Pelliniemi 1989; Kuopio et al. 1989a; Sharpe 1994; Haider et al. 1995). It is known that pericytes can disrupt their basement membrane and move away from the vessels (Sims 1991; Nehls and Drenckhahn 1993). Thus, newly formed Leydig cells may well possess basement membrane remnants of the continuous basal lamina of the vascular wall progenitor cells from which they arise (Huhtaniemi and Pelliniemi 1992; Haider et al. 1995). The existence of basement membrane remnants on the surface of young Leydig cells, therefore, supports the findings that Leydig cells derive from periendothelial pericytes.

7.4.3
Fetal-Like and Single-Spindle-Like Leydig Cells Are the First Leydig Cells That Appear During the Regeneration Process After EDS Administration in the Adult Rat Testis

In most previous publications, Leydig stem cells are described as elongated cells which express 3ß-hydroxysteroid dehydrogenase. As we showed, the pericytes do not express genes and products characteristic for the committed Leydig cells (Hardy et al. 1989; Mendis-Handagama and Ariyaratne 2001). This was confirmed at the molecular level by Ge et al. (2005, 2006) and Ge and Hardy (2007). The latter study, in addition, failed to establish gene expression similarity between the stem

Fig. 7.4 (continued) finally lose nestin, resulting in typical (yellow) Leydig cells (LC). Visualization of Leydig cells (**c**) and Leydig cell progenitors (pericytes) (**d**, *arrow*) in testes of transgenic mice expressing green fluorescent protein under the control of the nestin second-intron enhancer. T seminiferous tubules. **e** Demonstration of the transdifferentiation of pericytes into new Leydig cells at day 14 after EDS treatment. The cells of the clusters either coexpress nestin (*brown*) and CytP450scc (*blue*) or express CytP450scc only. **f** Colocalization of NF-H (*brown-black*) and vimentin (*blue*) in Leydig cells (*arrows*) and some Sertoli cells (*asterisks*) of the human testis (**c** – **e** ×330; **f** ×250). (**a** – **e** Modified from Davidoff et al. 2004)

Leydig cells and their late progeny. This shows that the cells expressing steroidogenic enzymes are not the Leydig stem cells but rather their descendants, differentiating through intermediate steps towards adult Leydig cells.

As demonstrated before, mural cells of the testis microvasculature are the stem/progenitor cells of the Leydig cells (Davidoff et al. 2004). This is true for both the intertubular and the peritubular Leydig stem/progenitor cells. These results are in accordance with the results obtained by Kerr et al. (1987b), investigating the perivascular origin of Leydig stem cells from mesenchymal cells. However, these authors defined the spindle-shaped or irregularly elongated interstitial cells as the precursors of morphologically recognizable Leydig cells. Furthermore, Kerr et al. (1987 b) found that 4 weeks after EDS treatment of rats, firstly a fetal-type Leydig cell population regenerates which showed a perivascular origin. This was followed by a population of peritubular origin. Another important result obtained by Kerr et al. (1987b) is that clusters of peritubular or perivascular Leydig cells were usually bordered by a thin wall of endothelial cytoplasm (probably the basement membrane), suggesting a close relationship between the newly formed Leydig cells and the testis vasculature. Surprisingly, O'Shaughnessy et al. (2008b) were not able to distinguish intertubular perivascular Leydig cell progenitors and adult Leydig cells in germ-cell-depleted rats (sterile rats, Molenaar et al. 1986b) after EDS administration. They described only peritubular progenitors without any relationship between these cells and the microvasculature. Moreover, the same authors observed a faster regeneration of new Leydig cells beginning at day 8 after EDS injection and explained this fact by the absence of germ cells. However, Kerr et al. (1987b) established the onset of Leydig cell regeneration between days 7 and 14 in rats with preserved germ cells. The reason for this apparent discrepancy remains unclear. The results obtained by Davidoff et al. (2004), analysing the process of regeneration of the neuroendocrine Leydig cells in EDS-treated rats (Kerr et al. 1987b), show that all new Leydig cells are descendants of stem/progenitor smooth muscle cells and pericytes of intertubular and peritubular vessels of the rat testis. Corresponding results were obtained during normal postnatal testis development. However, the distinct developmental stages of fetal-like, immature-adult and mature-adult populations of postnatal Leydig cells appeared to overlap partially. In accordance with Teerds and Rijntjes (2007), the individual Leydig cell populations could be easily recognized in EDS-treated rats, and numerous regenerating fetal-type Leydig cells were visible at day 14. It is important to note that even adult Leydig cells (postnatal day 60) retain their direct contacts with the blood vessels by means of long thin processes emerging from their perikarya (Fig. 5.3g, h).

7.4.4
Environmental Influences Are Responsible for the Diversity of Leydig Cell Phenotypes

There is increasing evidence that fetal and adult Leydig cells belong to the same cell lineage and have the same ancestor, and thus they are of common origin (Jackson et al. 1986; Kerr et al. 1988; Hardy et al. 1989; Davidoff et al. 1993, 1996, 2002, 2004; Middendorff et al. 1993; Sharpe 1994; Benton et al. 1995; Teerds et al. 1999; Müller et al. 2006; Park et al. 2007). In this regard, reports on the existence of so-called ectopic Leydig cells, or Leydig cells which are situated outside the testicular parenchyma, e.g. within the tunica albuginea, the spermatic cord (in association with peripheral nerves) as well as along the testicular vessels in the abdominal cavity (Watzka 1955; Peters 1977; Regadera et al. 1993; Sobhan-Sarbandi and Holstein 1988; Jeffs et al. 2001; Middendorff et al. 2002), are of major interest. Recent findings substantially support the existence of a common ancestor of all Leydig cell phenotypes (Davidoff et al. 2004). Thus, the phenotypic variability of Leydig cells probably results from local environmental or instructive influences acting upon the stem/progenitor Leydig cells and their descendants during different developmental, functional or pathological conditions in the testis (see Bixby et al. 2002 for the CNS). It is important to note that Leydig cells themselves express a great number of biologically active substances which are not only responsible for the autoregulation of their functions, but also influence the functions of the remaining testis structures in a paracrine fashion. Blood-borne factors, or factors released by endothelial cells, epithelial cells of seminiferous tubules or cells of the vessel wall seem to stimulate the occurrence of a fetal-type Leydig cell phenotype. In particular, decreases in testosterone levels after EDS application may affect the activity of stem-cell-like progenitors. It has been shown that cells of the microvasculature possess androgen receptors (Bergh and Damber 1992; Sharpe 1993, 1994; Ariyaratne and Mendis-Handagama 2000; Ariyaratne et al. 2000b), and that these receptors disappear after EDS-induced destruction of Leydig cells. Since biologically active factors such as testosterone, VEGF, NCAM, FGF2, nitric oxide and astrocyte-produced substances direct the commitment of stem/progenitor cells towards nerve and glial cells in the CNS, it is conceivable that analogous effects may also exist in the testis during Leydig cell generation. Some of these substances are also responsible for the blockage of the mitotic capability of stem/progenitor cells (Peunova and Enikolopov 1995; Amoureux et al. 2000). It has to be noted that most of the neuroactive factors mentioned above are expressed by Leydig cells or structural components of the testicular blood vessels.

7.5
EDS Treatment of Adult Rats Also Leads To Damage of the Seminiferous Epithelium

In addition to the effects on Leydig cells, EDS causes severe damage of the seminiferous epithelium (Jackson and Jackson 1984; Molenaar et al. 1985; Kerr et al. 1988; Sharpe 1994; Bakalska et al. 2001; 2004, 2006; Atanassova et al. 2006; Yang et al. 2006), in particular affecting spermatogenesis (loss of elongated spermatids, disappearance of round spermatids and pachytene spermatocytes) with maximum changes detectable around day 14 after EDS administration (Bartlett et al. 1986). As mentioned already, the number of progenitor Leydig cells that transform into adult-type Leydig cells remarkably increased around days 20-22 after EDS administration (Teerds et al. 1999). The fact that these cells accumulate around tubules with impaired spermatogenesis suggests that Sertoli-cell- or germ-cell-derived factors promote the increase in number and activity of adult-type Leydig cells (Kerr and Sharpe 1985; Paniagua et al. 1988; Sharpe 1993, 1994; Teerds 1996). High concentrations of testosterone were shown to be necessary for maintenance of pachytene spermatocytes (Haider et al. 1990; Neumann et al. 1993), and especially for the transformation of round spermatids into elongated ones (Haider 1988; Bartlett et al. 1989a; Haider et al. 1990; Ariyaratne and Mendes-Handagama 2000; Schäfers et al. 2001). It is known that Leydig cell numbers can change in adult species depending on the stages of spermatogenesis (Kerr et al. 1993; Paniagua et al. 1988). In addition, there is strong evidence for a narrow relationship between Leydig cells and Sertoli cells with respect to the regulation of their number and functional activity (Sharpe 1994).

7.6
The Pericyte Is a Peculiar Cell Type Just Now Beginning To Be Understood

The discovery that the testicular Leydig cells originate from microvascular pericytes justifies a short characterization of this very interesting cell population.

7.6.1
Pericytes and Vascular Smooth Muscle Cells Are of the Same Cell Lineage

The pericytes represent one of the main components of the vascular wall. They reside on the adluminal site in a vascular niche consisting of endothelial cells, the basement membrane and enveloping periendothelial cells (von Ebner 1971; termed "pericytes" by Zimmermann 1923). In addition to their common embedding in the basement membrane (Meyrick and Reid 1979; Bergers and Song 2005), pericytes and endothelial cells are interconnected at some sites by different cell-to-cell contacts (Hirschi and D'Amore 1996; Sims 1986; Hayden et al. 2008).

The testis contains a dense vascular network with a prominent microvascular portion. Microvessels of the testis are situated within intertubular columns, the lamina propria and the peritubular spaces of interstitial connective tissue (Weerasooriya and Yamamoto 1985; Murakami et al. 1989; Setchell et al. 1994; Ergün et al. 1994a, b; 1996; Zengin et al. 2006). Large vessels also contain subendothelial pericytes (Andreeva et al. 1998). Microvessels generally contain two cell types, namely endothelial cells and vascular smooth muscle cells/pericytes. Towards the smallest branches of the microvasculature, the midcapillaries, the vascular smooth muscle cells, which lie perpendicularly (circularly) to the longitudinal axis and tend to encircle the endothelial tubes, gradually become elongated pericytes which are mainly oriented longitudinally to the vessel direction (Sims 1991; Nehls and

Drenckhahn 1993). The results of the study of Davidoff et al. (2004) showed that there is essential similarity between the pericytes and the smooth muscle cells of the testis microvasculature. According to Alliot et al. (1999), pericytes and vascular smooth muscle cells are of common origin in brain parenchymal vessels (Hayden et al. 2008; da Silva Meirelles et al. 2008).

7.6.2
Several Marker Antigens Characterize Pericytes and Smooth Muscle Cells of the Adult Rat Testis Microvasculature

Pericytes and vascular smooth muscle cells are largely defined and identified on the basis of their location and shape (Thomas 1999). Pericytes in different locations of the body show certain differences in the expression of marker substances (Morikawa et al. 2002). Generally, the following markers were found in pericytes: αSMA, non-muscle mosin, tropomyosin, desmin, nestin, PDGFR-ß, aminopeptidase A, aminopeptidase N (CD13), antigen 3G5 and NG2.

In the rat testis, in addition to the structures described by Fröjdman et al. (1997), during normal testis development and after EDS administration in adult rats, nestin immunoreactivity was associated with non-endothelial cells of blood vessel walls of the testicular microvasculature in the smooth muscle cells of intertubular arterioles, large and small capillaries and venules as well as in pericytes of smaller peritubular capillaries and large venules (Davidoff et al. 2004). The nestin-immunoreactive vascular wall cells of the testis also contained αSMA and to a lesser extent desmin. Detection of NG2, PDGFR-ß and PDGFR-α in these cells provided additional arguments for their stem-cell-like nature (Davidoff et al. 2004). NG2, a chondroitin sulphate proteoglycan, is the rat analogue (the murine one is AN2) of the human melanoma proteoglycan, also termed "high molecular weight melanoma-associated antigen", whose specific extracellular matrix ligands are collagen V and VI. There is strong evidence that NG2 is localized to activated blood vessel vascular smooth muscle cells and pericytes (Ozerdem et al. 2001) besides its expression by neural and glial cell progenitors of the central and peripheral nervous system (Schneider et al. 2001; Belachew et al. 2003). Vascular smooth muscle cells/pericytes express both αSMA and NG2 (Darland and D'Amore (2001) (Fig.7.1e, f). As mentioned earlier, PDGF-B- and PDGFR-ß-deficient mice show formation of blood vessels lacking pericytes and vascular smooth muscle cells (Lindahl et al. 1997a, b; Hellström et al. 2001; Basciani et al. 2002; Lindblom et al. 2003), and RGS5 gene, a member of the RGS family of GTPase-activating proteins, which was characterized as a new marker protein of vascular smooth muscle cell and pericytes is downregulated in these mice models (Bondjers et al. 2003; Cho et al. 2003). In vascular smooth muscle cells and pericytes, Davidoff et al. (2004) recognized also FGF2, PDGFR-ß, the proteoglycan NG2 and NF-H immunoreactivity. Some of these substances (NG2 and PDGFR-ß) were also found to be expressed transiently in newly arising progenitor Leydig cells (Fig. 7.4i, l). These results provide further evidence that the pericytes represent the stem/progenitor cells of the Leydig cell lineage.

7.6.3
Pericytes Are Stem/Progenitor Cells

Angiogenesis, the collective term for the sprouting, splitting, growth and remodelling of blood vessels, is a central process in vertebrate embryonic development. Angiogenesis consists of the endothelial cell sprouting and the maturation process of recruitment of mural (pericytes and smooth muscle) cells - smooth muscle cells for large vessels and pericytes for the microvasculature. The mural cells, directly lining vascular endothelial cells, are called "periendothelial cells", whereas cells of the other layers are called "perivascular cells". The endothelial cells, the periendothelial pericytes and the smooth muscle cells are components of the intima of blood vessels. The term "perivascular cell" is used for the vascular media (smooth muscle cells and connective tissue cells and fibres) and the various structural components of the vascular adventitia.

Pericytes are a heterogeneous cell population, and until now there is no common marker by which they can be distinguished unequivocally from all other cell types (Bondjers et al. 2006). By culturing mouse embryonic stem cells on OP9 stromal cells, Lindskog et al. (2006) showed that OP9 cells induce differentiation of embryonic stem cells to pericytes that had first differentiated into endothelial cells. These authors found that the induction of pericyte marker genes is temporally separated from the induction of smooth muscle cell genes, and does not require PDGF-B or TGF-ß$_1$ signalling. It seems likely that PDGF-B is not responsible for pericyte differentiation but for their proliferation and recruitment into certain tissues (e.g. CNS components). In addition, embryonic stem cell derived sprouts recruit vascular smooth muscle cells/pericytes from cocultured mouse embryonic hepatocyte growth factor (HGF) fibroblasts. Recent studies provide evidence that the HGF, expressed by endothelial cells, may mediate angiopoietin-induced smooth muscle/pericyte cell recruitment, and Ang1 and Ang2 were shown to exert opposing effects on the HGF (Kobayashi et al. 2006). In addition to the commonly used markers for pericytes (αSMA, desmin, NG2, RGS5 and PDGFR-ß), Bondjers et al. (2006) recently revealed three new ones in the CNS, namely the ATP-sensitive potassium channel (Kir6.1), the sulphonylurea receptor 2 (SUR2B) and the putative Notch receptor ligand delta homologue 1 (DLK1).

Pericyte differentiation is locally regulated and dependent on heterotypic cell contacts such as gap junctions, peg-and-socket junctions and adhesion plaques (Rucker et al. 2000; Hayden et al. 2008). Allt and Lawrenson (2001) found that growth factors and extracellular matrix molecules modulate phenotype and function of pericytes. Furthermore, αSMA and NG2, expressed by pericytes, increase in pericyte precursors in response to TGF-ß$_1$ treatment and in response to their contact with endothelial cells (Rucker et al. 2000; Darland and D'Amore 2001; Darland et al. 2003). Using VEGF-LacZ transgenic mice, Darland et al. (2003) demonstrated VEGF expression by NG2-positive pericytes as well as astrocytes in the developing retinal vasculature. Moreover, neural stem cells and neural crest stem cells are able to differentiate into smooth muscle cells (Galli et al. 2000; Rietze et al. 2001; Oishi et al. 2002; Le Douarin et al. 2008). In the adult skeletal muscle, progenitors have been found to be generated by either mesenchymal or neural stem cells (Bailey et al. 2001). Recent findings show that the adventitia in aortic roots harboured large numbers of cells expressing stem cell markers, and under the influence of PDGF-BB these cells may differentiate into smooth muscle cells (Hu et al. 2004; Hoofnagle et al. 2004).

The results obtained by Davidoff et al. (2004) provide unequivocal evidence that the stem cell progenitors of the Leydig cells are pericytes and smooth muscle cells, which reside in the wall of the testicular microvasculature. These data show for the first time that progenitor cells with neuroendocrine characteristics are homed in the wall of blood vessels and that the vessel wall represents the niche for Leydig cell progenitors. It is well documented that stem/progenitor cells of cells which possess mesodermal progeny can reside in the wall of blood vessels (De Angelis et al. 1999; Minasi et al. 2002; Sampoalesi et al. 2003; da Silva Meirelles et al. 2008). There is also evidence that muscle-derived stem cells first attach to capillaries of the muscles and then participate in regeneration after muscle damage (Torrente et al. 2001).

7.6.4
Pericytes and Multipotent Mesenchymal Stem/Stromal Cells in Diverse Human and Rodent Tissues Comprise Mural and Perivascular Cells

Pericytes play important roles in the control of angiogenesis and the stabilization of vessels (Hirshi and D'Amore 1996; Lindahl et al. 1997b; Hess et al. 2004; Hayden et al. 2008). A lot of evidence suggests that pericytes are disseminated as stem cells throughout an organism. This leads to the presumption that pericytes are the true stem cells that comprise the mesenchymal stem cells of the body (Bianco et al. 2001; da Silva Meirelles et al. 2008). Here some examples.

The bone marrow, in addition to the well-described haematopoietic stem cells, contains a heterogeneous population of non-haematopoietic stem cells, including some very rare cell populations (e.g. multipotent adult progenitor cells, marrow-isolated adult multilineage inducible cells, multipotent adult stem cells as well as epiblast-derived very small embryonic-like stem cells) that displays several features of pluripotent stem cells with the ability to differentiate into cells from all three germ layers (Ratajczak et al. 2008). The very small embryonic-like stem cells and the SSEA-1 mesenchymal stem cells are thought to be the most primitive progenitors in the murine bone marrow mesenchymal compartment (Anjos-Afonso and Bonnet 2007; Ratajczak et al. 2008). One of the members of the non-haematopoietic stem cells is the stromal cells that reside on the abluminal aspects of marrow sinusoids, thus representing in fact perivascular cells and resembling smooth muscle cells and pericytes of other organs (Bianco and Robey 2000). In this respect, Bianco and Cossu (1999) presumed that microvascular districts may represent the specific niche where multipotent progenitors are retained in adult tissues (De Angelis et al. 1999; Minasi et al. 2000). Also the so-called perivascular reticular cells (Sugiyama et al. 2006; Kiel and Morrison 2006) were shown to expand between the bone marrow vasculature and the bone matrix and to be of osteoblast lineage (Rouleau et al. 1990). There are findings providing direct evidence that pericytes in situ serve as a reservoir of primitive precursor cells capable of giving rise to cells of multiple lineages, including osteoblasts, chondrocytes, adipocytes and fibroblasts (Doherty et al. 1998). As discussed above, the bone marrow reticular cells (also referred to as "bone mesenchymal stem cells") are pericytes in nature and may transdifferentiate into osteoblasts and chondroblasts and acquire neuronal characteristics (Tomasek et al. 2002; Towler 2003; Tropel et al. 2006; Anjos-Afonso and Bonnet 2007).

Hepatic stem cells (hepatic progenitor cells; Mancino et al. 2007) are resident hepatic cells located at the levels of the canals of Herring, near the portal spaces (Dabeva et al. 1993; Theise et al. 1999; Saxena and Theise 2004). On the bais of distinctive morphological features in different mammals, including humans, they are designated as oval cells, small hepatocytes, hepatic progenitor cells, or "intermediate hepatocyte-like cells" (Mancino et al. 2007).

The hepatic stellate cells are also considered to be liver-specific pericytes (Sato et al. 2003; Lee et al. 2007; Cassiman et al. 2007). These cells are characterized by myocyte-specific properties (desmin and αSMA) and express in addition neural markers such as nerve growth factor, brain-derived neurotrophic factor, neurotrophin-3, neurotrophin-4/neurotrophin-5, p75, TrkB, TrkC, synaptophysin, GFAP and NCAM (Niki et al. 1999; Cassiman et al. 1999, 2001, 2002; Sato et al. 2003; Roskams et al. 2004). In addition, hepatic stellate cells were shown to be able to transdifferentiate towards transitional cells (intermediate between hepatic stellate cells and myofibroblasts) and myofibroblasts (Cassiman et al. 2002). The hepatic oval stem cells can transdifferentiate into neural cells in the neonatal mouse brain (Deng et al. 2003; Mancino et al. 2007). There are some similarities between hepatic oval stem cells and haematopoietic progenitor cells, but the bone marrow progenitors are not the source of expanding oval cells in injured liver (Menthena et al. 2004). In addition, a mixed epithelial/mesenchymal oval stem cell population capable of repopulating injured rat liver was recently described by Yovchev et al. (2008). Notably, following transplantation of pancreatic epithelial progenitor cells into rat liver, these cells differentiate into hepatocytes, thereby demonstrating similarity between the progenitor cells of both organs (Dabeva et al. 1997).

These results allow the presumption that a more widespread system of somatic stem cells than thought before exists within an organism. Although a large number of common genes were found in stem cells of various body regions or organs, there are also genes which are exclusively expressed in certain organs (Ramalho-Santos et al. 2002). On the basis of gene analyses, Romalho-Santos et al. (2002) established that neural stem cells are more similar to embryonic stem cells, whereas haematopoietic stem cells are more similar to the main stem cell population of the bone marrow.

Neural stem cells were found to be characterized by a close relationship to brain blood vessels (Palmer et al. 2000). However, the brain stem cells, also referred to as "neuroepithelial stem cells", are not a structural component of the vascular wall, but generate proliferative clusters, consisting of neural progenitors, committed neuroblasts and glial and endothelial precursors (Rao 2004a). In contrast to the testis, the neural stem cells are found in the vicinity of brain capillaries, and their development is influenced by signals provided by the out-sprouting capillary endothelial cells (Palmer et al. 2000). In addition, a common multipotent neuroepithelial stem cell type which can differentiate into most major types of cells in the CNS and the peripheral nervous system was described by Mujtaba et al. (1998). Importantly, the existence of a common neurohaematopoietic stem cell in the human brain has also been revealed by Shih et al. (2001).

Dore-Duffy et al. (2006) emphasized the multipotential characteristics of pericytes in the nervous system on the basis of their neural characteristics and their capability to produce neurons and glia (astrocytes and oligodendrocytes). Pericytes of the CNS are nestin/NG2-positive and, during neurogenesis or activation, αSMA-positive. CNS pericytes also have macrophage qualities during brain injury (Balabanov et al. 1996). In response to traumatic brain injury, approximately 40% of rat brain pericytes can migrate out of the vascular wall into the perivascular neuropil (Dore-Duffy et al. 2000).

Moreover, Yamashima et al. (2004), using different methodical approaches essentially including electron-microscopic immunohistochemistry, revealed that neural progenitors during ischaemia in the hippocampal subgranular zone (SGZ) of the dentate gyrus of Japanese monkeys (Macaca fuscata) are generated by pericytes of capillaries and/or adventitial cells of arterioles (called "vascular adventitia").

In the adult human pancreas, enriched non-endocrine epithelial cells generate pancreatic islet progenitor cells (D'Alessandro et al. 2007). Moreover, Lardon et al. (2002) found nestin immunoreactivity in the pancreas primarily as marker for reactive stellate cells, pericytes (Alliot et al. 1999) or endothelial cells during active angiogenesis. Stellate cells were also positive for desmin, vimentin, and GFAP (Apte et al. 2007; Bachem et al. 1998; Niki et al. 1999). Stellate cells are able to transdifferentiate into myofibroblast-like cells under pathological conditions. These results were partially confirmed by Klein et al. (2003), who established in the adult human pancreas that nestin is expressed in vascular endothelial cells located adjacent to the duct epithelium where endocrine differentiation occurs as well as in islet cells and in the exocrine pancreas. Considering the intricacy necessary to discriminate between endothelial cells and pericytes in small blood vessels (capillaries) by fluorescence microscopy (Lammert et al. 2001), the strict assignment of the nestin-positive cells to endothelial cells might be challenged. Moreover, Kruse et al. (2004, 2006 b) showed that pancreatic stellate-like cells have the capacity of self-renewal and can differentiate spontaneously into phenotypes of all three germ layers with marker proteins for neurons, glial cells, epithelial cells, chondrocytes, smooth muscle cells and secretory cells (insulin- and amylase-producing). Recently, Kajahn et al. (2008) established that both human pancreas- and skin-derived stem/progenitor cells demonstrate patterns of differentiation across lineage boundaries into cell types of normally ectodermal, mesodermal and entodermal origin. Pluripotent pericytes of the pancreas are also involved in islet and microcirculation remodelling (Hayden et al. 2008). The latter study, in addition, provided evidence that pericytes might be capable of forming closed capillary tubes, a novel finding of presumed importance for certain pathophysiological events in the pancreas. Close association of pancreatic microvascular nestin-positive cells and endocrine islet cells has been established by Treutelaar et al. (2003).

The mesangial cells of the kidney seem to have a haematopoietic cell origin, a process that does not involve cell fusion (Masuya et al. 2003). Renal mesangial cells express VEGF and Flt-1 (Takahashi et al. 1995). Flt-1 is an endothelium-specific receptor for VEGF, and its gene expression is upregulated upon stimulation by PDGF. Moreover, VEGF receptors were found in podocytes and mesangial cells of human kidneys (Amemiya et al. 1999; Thomas et al. 2000).

Pericyte progenitor cells could also be isolated from the aortic wall (Howson et al. 2005). These spheroid-forming cells were positive for NG2, nestin, Tie2, PDGFR-α, and PDGFR-ß. A multipotent, self-renewing cell population that originates from the dorsal aorta was called "mesoangioblasts". The corresponding cells were able to differentiate into most mesodermal tissues (Minasi et al. 2002). Apparently, these cells also supply the vasculature with endothelial cells and pericytes. On the other hand, angiohaematopoietic cells migrate from the paraaortic splanchnopleura into the ventral wall of the aorta, where they differentiate into haemogenic endothelial cells and haematopoietic cells (Tavian et al. 2005).

Skin stem cells reside in the adult hair follicle, sebaceous gland, and epidermis (Waters et al. 2007; Fuchs 2008). Skin-derived precursors are located within follicular dermal papillae and are capable of producing neural and mesodermal progeny and possess a neural crest origin (Paus et al. 2008). The skin-derived precursors are also immunoreactive for nestin during development and retain their multipotency until adulthood (Fernandes et al. 2008). In the bulge region of the hair follicle, multipotent epithelial stem cell types were established (Sieber-Blum and Grim 2004a, b; Ohyama 2007). A new multipotent stem cell population was described by Mignone et al. (2007) which can give rise to neurosphere-like structures that differentiate into neuronal, astrocytic, oligodendrocytic, smooth muscle, adipocytic and other phenotypes (see also Wiese et al. 2004; Yu et al. 2006; Kruse et al. 2006a). A relationship between these stem cells and the vasculature of the skin has been established (Amoh et al. 2004, 2005a, b; Chang et al. 2002).

Recently, dental pulp and periodontal ligament stem cells were isolated (Liu et al. 2006). These cells are located within a microvascular niche and possess self-renewal and multilineage (adipogenic and neural) capabilities (Gronthos et al. 2002). Dental pulp stem cells as well as human bone marrow stromal stem cells behave as pericytes and express the marker 3G5 as well as αSMA and CD146 (Shi and Gronthos 2003).

Skeletal muscle stem cells, the satellite cells, are quiescent cells that reside under the basal lamina of muscle fibres (Zammit et al. 2006; Day et al. 2007) and represent the main source for myoblasts in postnatal muscle. They are a heterogenous cell population composed of stem cells and committed progenitors (Kuang et al. 2007). Muscle satellite cells are multipotent stem cells that exhibit myogenic, osteogenic and adipogenic differentiation activity (Asakura et al. 2001). Skeletal muscle stem cells also possess a close relationship with cells of the vessel wall (endothelial cells and pericytes) (De Angelis et al. 1999; Tavian et al. 2005; Péault et al. 2007). However, pericytes of human skeletal muscle are myogenic precursors distinct from satellite cells (Dellavalle et al. 2007), reinforcing the important role of pericytes as stem/progenitor cells for repair of damaged skeletal muscle cells. Muscle stem cells show plasticity. Skeletal-muscle-derived stem cells (side-population stem cells, muscle-derived stem cells and mesoangioblasts) can give rise, after transplantation, to myogenic, vascular (pericytes, vascular smooth muscle cells and endothelial cells) and neural (Schwann) cells as well as contribute to the synchronized reconstruction of blood vessels, muscle fibres and peripheral nerves (Tamaki et al. 2005). Under conditions of high glucose concentrations, muscle-derived stem cells differentiate into adipocytes (Aguiari et al. 2008).

Different stem cell types were identified in the postnatal heart (cardiac stem cells, progenitors, precursors and amplifying cells), which most probably reflects subsequent steps during the progressive evolution from a more primitive to a more differentiated phenotype (Anversa et al. 2006a, b, 2007; Bearzi et al. 2007). There is a very close relationship between vasculogenesis/angiogenesis and cardiomyocyte development by cardiac stem cells (Kajstura et al. 2008; Tillmanns et al. 2008). Recently, a new cell type was found in the juvenile mouse ventricle (not in atrium) that was classified as mesoangioblast (Galvez et al. 2008). These cardiac mesoangioblasts express both endothelial and pericyte markers and spontaneously differentiate into spontaneously contracting cardiomyocytes.

There is strong evidence for a neural crest origin of the thymus perivascular mesenchyme, which represents vessel-associated pericytes along the entire thymus vasculature (Müller et al. 2008). As further revealed, not only the pericytes, but also smooth muscle cells of the embryonic and adult thymus are of neural crest origin (Foster et al. 2008). Neural-crest-derived cells invade the thymus before day 13.5 of embryonic development and differentiate into smooth muscle cells associated with large vessels and pericytes associated with capillaries. These cells remain associated with the vasculature until adulthood.

Our results thus support the idea that during development stem cells use blood vessel formation and their invasive growth into different organ anlages (Ivanova and Lammert 2003), and remain within the adult organs for purposes of physiological turnover and pathological or experimental repair, as well as for cell number increase during some processes such as cell hyperplasia and tumorigenesis (Minasi et al. 2002; Bianco and Robey 2000). Depending on their final location, these stem/progenitor cells seem to be influenced by local factors and change some of their primary qualities as this was evidenced for the neural (crest) stem cells in adult organs (Lothian and Lendahl 1997; Clarke et al. 2000; Galli et al. 2000; Shihabuddin et al. 2000; Kruger et al. 2002; Song et al. 2002; Rajan et al. 2003).

Recently, a proposal for the nomenclature of mesenchymal stem cells of nearly all organs of the body was developed by the International Society for Cellular Therapy (Horwitz et al. 2005). According to this statement, mesenchymal stem cells in culture should be designated as "multipotential mesenchymal stromal cells", whereas the term "mesenchymal stem cells" should be reserved for cells from primary tissues that can produce colony forming unit fibroblasts in vitro and can repopulate tissues with multilineage capacity of differentiation in vivo. There are a large number of different mesenchymal stem/stromal cells, which include bone marrow stromal stem cells, bone marrow mesenchymal stem cells, side-population stem cells, stellate and oval cells of the liver, myofibroblasts, skeletal muscle, blood mesnechymal stem cells, vascular wall mesenchymal stem cells, testicular mesenchymal stem cells, cardiac mesenchymal stem cells, pancreatic mesenchymal stem cells, and skin and kidney mesenchymal stem cells (see da Silva Meirelles et al. 2008, for a review).

Mesenchymal stem/stromal cells are self-renewing cells that can give rise to mesodermally derived tissues including bone, cartilage, muscle, stromal cells, tendon, and connective tissue. Cultured mesenchymal stem cells are well characterized, plastic-adherent, spindle-shaped cells that express a panel of key markers, including CD105 (endoglein, SH2), CD73 (ecto-5 nucleotidase, SH3, SH4), CD166 (ALCAM), CD29 ($ß_1$-integrin), CD44 (H-CAM), CD90 (Thy-1) and STRO-1 (Bühring et al. 2007). Depending on their source (e.g. bone marrow or placenta) and on culture conditions, mesenchymal stem cells additionally express CD349 (fizzed-9), SSEA-4, Oct-4, nanog-3, and nestin (Battula et al. 2008). Multipotential human adipose-derived stromal stem cells exhibit a perivascular phenotype (expression of STRO-1, CD146 and 3G5 in vitro and in vivo), providing evidence for the close relationship between the human adipose tissue and the pericytes (Zannettino et al. 2007b).

7.6.5
Mesenchymal/Stromal Stem Cells Possess Remarkable Plasticity

Rajantie et al. (2004) showed that bone-marrow-derived cells participate in angiogenesis and can differentiate into vascular mural cells (pericytes). Furthermore, myeloid lineage progenitors can give rise to vascular endothelium (Bailey et al. 2006), and multipotent adult progenitor cells from bone marrow can differentiate into functional hepatocyte-like cells (Schwartz et al. 2002). Cells infused at bone marrow transplantation contribute to skeletal muscle myoblasts and endothelium and acquire properties of hepatic, biliary duct, lung, gut and skin epithelia as well as of neuroectoderm and a cardiac myoblast phenotype (Jiang et al. 2003). Neural stem cells may repopulate the haematopoietic system (Bjornson et al. 1999). On the other hand, haematopoietic stem cells also possess cardiomyogenic potential (Jackson et al. 2001). Moreover, stem cells (muscle satellite cells, which reside between the sarcolemma and the basal lamina of the muscle fibre) from murine skeletal muscle transplanted into irradiated mice contributed to the regeneration of the entire haematopoietic system (Jackson et al. 1999). Human stem cells isolated from adult skeletal muscle were able to differentiate into neural phenotypes. Meyrick and Reid (1978) have shown that under hypoxic stress pericytes of the lung microvasculature have the capability to develop into smooth muscle cells. Bone marrow multipotent adult progenitor cells give rise to mesenchymal lineage cells, endothelium, endoderm, all types of brain cells and all somatic cells after injection into the blastocyst (Jiang et al. 2003, 2004). Hippocampal stem cells from adult mice can differentiate into neural crest derivatives such as melanocytes, chondocytes and smooth muscle cells (Alexanian and Sieber-Blum 2003).

Bone-marrow-derived mesenchymal stem cells can generate bone and associated bone marrow structures upon subcutaneous transplantation in vivo. A bone marrow operating system, which represents niches containing haematopoietic cells, is developed during such processes (Miura et al. 2006). In this regard, Dominici et al. (2004) established that haematopoietic cells and osteoblasts are derived from a common progenitor after bone marrow transplantation. Recently, in addition to existing mesenchymal stem cells and precursors of adipocyte and endothelial cells, cells involved in haematopoietic activity were revealed in the stromal vascular fraction of adult human adipose tissue (Miñana et al. 2008).

Pericytes as well as vascular smooth muscle cells behave as multipotent cells and can transform into osteoblasts, smooth muscle cells, chondroblasts and preadipocytes (Sims 1991). Transition of pericytes towards periendothelial smooth muscle cells occurred under hypoxic stress and during angiogenesis (Meyrick and Reid 1978; Sims 1991; Nehls and Drenckhahn 1993; Hirschi and D'Amore 1996; Thomas 1999). In brain, parenchyma vessels, pericytes and periendothelial smooth muscle cells coexpress aminopeptidase N, aminopeptidase A and nestin, which permits the conclusion that both cell types are of common origin (Alliot et al. 1999). Ehler et al. (1995) showed that pericytes of intact microvessels possess a pattern of protein expression characteristic of smooth muscle cells, thus confirming the close relationship between smooth muscle cells and pericytes. In this respect, a new embryonic vascular precursor cell that gives rise to both main vascular cell types was revealed by Yamashita et al. (2000). This precursor cell can differentiate into endothelial cells under the influence of VEGF, whereas PDGF-BB promotes its differentiation into vascular smooth muscle cells and pericytes (Carmeliet 2000; Holmgren et al. 1991; Hirschi et al. 1999; Helström et al. 2001). Finally, brain pericytes and vascular smooth muscle cells have been shown to have a common neuroectodermal origin (Korn et al. 2002). The results obtained by Davidoff et al. (2004) confirm the common lineage of both cell types, showing that both are stem-cell-like progenitors of Leydig cells. In addition, both cell types proliferate after EDS administration (self-renewing), and possess immunoreactivity for the specific markers for pericytes/smooth muscle cells and stem cells, i.e. nestin, αSMA, NG2 and PDGFR-ß.

As discussed above, stem Leydig cells and Leydig cell progenitors resemble to a large extent adult stem cells (Weissman 2000; Beauchamp et al. 2000; Anderson 2001; Ramalho-Santos et al. 2002; Jiang et al. 2002; Danet et al. 2002; Herzog et al. 2003). Adult stem cells have been found in various tissues, including bone marrow (Bianco and Robey 2000; Woodbury et al. 2002; Matsuoka et al. 2001), CNS (McKay 1997; Rietze et al. 2001; Gritti et al. 2002; Okano 2002a, b; Clarke et al. 2000; Bjornson et al. 1999), peripheral nervous system (Morrison et al. 1999), skeletal and smooth muscle (Ferrari et al. 1998; Jackson et al. 1999; Majka et al. 2003; De Angelis et al. 1999; Nadin et al. 2003; Torrente et al. 2001; Tamaki et al. 2002, 2003; Qu-Petersen et al. 2002; Hirschi and Majesky 2004), adult myocardium (Oh et al. 2003), aorta (Howson et al. 2005), umbilical veins (Ishisaki et al. 2003; Marcus and Woodbury 2008), vena cava (da Silva Meirelles 2006), small vessels from kidney glomeruli, brain, spleen, liver, lung, bone marrow, muscle, thymus and pancreas (Zulewski et al. 2001; Shu et al. 2002; da Silva Meirelles et al. 2006), intestine (Bixby et al. 2002; Kruger et al. 2002; Bondurand et al. 2003), liver (Petersen et al. 1999, 2003; Lagasse et al. 2000; Deng et al. 2003; Wang et al. 2001, 2003; Wulf et al. 2003), pancreas (Hunziker and Stein 2000; Zulewski et al. 2001; Lechner et al. 2002; Yang et al. 2002), skin (Slack 2000; Toma et al. 2001; Blanpain and Fuchs 2006), thymus (Botham et al. 2001), exfoliated human deciduous teeth (Miura et al. 2003), testis (Lo et al. 2004; Davidoff et al. 2004; Ge et al. 2006) and retina (Turner and Cepko 1987). In these tissues, stem cells are thought to replenish cells that are lost by physiological turnover or following pathological conditions including injury and degenerative diseases (Okano 2002a, b).

Most of these adult stem cells are multipotent and possess the capability to transform under conditions such as tissue injury, cell culturing, intra-arterial transport and direct transplantation into cells with neuroectodermal (neurons and glia) and mesodermal (endothelial cells, cardiomyocytes, smooth muscle cells, osteocytes, chondrocytes, adipocytes and renal tubule epithelium cells) characteristics (Toma et al. 2001; Krause et al. 2001; Zulewski et al. 2001; Deng et al. 2003; Kale et al. 2003; Torrente et al. 2001; LaBarge and Blau 2002; Miura et al. 2003; Syder et al. 2004; da Silva Meirelles et al. 2006, 2008). Also, a large population of vascular progenitor cells in the adventitia can differentiate into smooth muscle cells, thereby contributing to development of atherosclerosis (Hu et al. 2004). Generally, there is growing evidence for a close relationship between mesenchymal stem cells and pericytes (Doherty et al. 1998; Farrington-Rock et al. 2004), and in certain publications, pericytes may have been misinterpreted as endothelial cells because of their extremely close proximity (Rajantie et al. 2004).

Before the recent identification of smooth muscle cells and pericytes as the Leydig cell progenitors (Davidoff et al. 2004), only a few publications considered pericytes as potential progenitors for the Leydig cells. Morphological investigations by Jackson et al. (1986) suggested that Leydig cells arise by differentiation from a pool of connective tissue cells that included fibroblasts, lymphatic endothelial cells and pericytes. Furthermore, Russell et al. (1995) published electron-microscopic data from developing rats (up to 20 days of age) indicating mitotic figures in undifferentiated perivascular fibroblast-like cells at low frequency, and the authors presumed that these cells could represent Leydig cell progenitors. According to Russel et al. (1995), these cells appeared to share characteristics of pericytes.

7.7
The Vascular Stem Cell Niche and the Stem-Cell-Like Progenitors of Testicular Leydig Cells

Vascular stem cell niches are local tissue microenvironments that are generated by endothelial cells and/or further mural cells as well as other non-vascular cells that maintain resident stem cells and regulate their properties. The stem cell niche is also important for harbouring of stem cells in a quiescent state (Nishikawa and Osawa 2006). A common feature of this niche is to provide a basement membrane to cells that are unable to form their own membrane. The basement membrane contains laminins, collagen IV and fibronectin (Nikolova et al. 2006a, b; Morrison and Spradling 2008; da Silva Meirelles et al. 2008).

In the CNS, a close relationship was established between neurogenesis and vasculogenesis (angiogenesis). The vascular niche in the CNS comprises stem and endothelial cells of the brain microvasculature that contribute to the generation of extravascular nodules in which new nerve cells differentiate under the influence of intrinsic or/and externally released factors (Palmer et al. 2000; Louissaint et al. 2002). In contrast, the close relationship between stem-cell-like progenitors and the microvasculature of the testis established by Davidoff et al. (2004) shows an essential difference, namely that the non-endothelial Leydig cell progenitors are an integral structural component of the vessel walls (Shi and Gronthos 2003; mesenchymal stem cell populations reside in the microvasculature of their tissue of origin). Endothelial cells of the microvasculature of the testis were nestin- and αSMA-negative. We cannot exclude a role of the endothelial cells in the activation of vascular smooth muscle cells and pericytes. In contrast to the CNS, however, endothelial cells were not seen within the nodules of newly formed Leydig cells.

Zhao et al. (2008) recently established that proliferating cells and putative neural progenitors in both the subgranular zone (SGZ) and the subventricular zone (SVZ) are closely associated with the vasculature, indicating that factors released from blood vessels may have a direct impact on adult neural progenitors (Mercier et al. 2002; Alvarez-Buylla and Lim 2004; Palmer et al. 2000). In apparent support of such a view, infusion of VEGF promotes in a VEGF-receptor-dependent manner cell proliferation in the SGZ and the SVZ (Cao et al. 2004).

It is now well established that the astroglial lineage provides multipotent neural stem cells (Ihrie and Alvarez-Buylla 2008). Astrocytic neural stem cells are part of a developmental lineage extending from neuroepithelium to radial glia and germinal astrocytes (Doetsch et al. 1999a, b, 2003b; Alvarez-Buylla and Garcia Verdugo 2002; Ihrie and Alvarez-Buylla 2008). Alvarez-Builla and Lim (2004) showed (1) that astrocytes can serve as both stem cells and niche cells, (2) that a basal lamina and concomitant vasculogenesis may be essential or at least supportive for the niche and (3) that "embryonic" molecular morphogens and signals persist in these niches, playing a critical role during adult neurogenesis. SVZ astrocytes (type B cells) are in intimate contact with other SVZ cell types, including the rapidly dividing transit amplifying (type C) cells and the committed migratory neuroblasts (type A cells). B cells presumably act as self-renewing primary precursors of both type C and type A cells. B and C cells cultured in serum-free medium in direct contact with monolayers of astrocytes proliferate to form colonies of young neurons (Lim and Alvarez-Buylla 1999). Similarly, astroglial-derived soluble and membrane-bound factors promote the proliferation and neuronal fate of hippocampal stem cells (Song et al. 2002).

During development and in regenerative tissues, stem cell maintenance and differentiation are frequently dependent on the closeness of a basal lamina. In the SVZ, B cells have the most extensive contact with the basal lamina of the pial layer.

In the adult brain, a close relationship between vasculogenesis and neurogenesis exists (Louissaint et al. 2002). Brain blood vessels in the SVZ are intimately associated with the basal lamina (Mercier et al. 2002), and the basal lamina is interdigitated with astrocytes that function as both stem and niche cells. In the SGZ, clusters of endothelial cell division are spatially and temporally related to clusters of neurogenesis (Palmer et al. 2000). VEGF receptors are detectable in these clusters of cell division. Intraventricular infusion of VEGF increases proliferation of both SVZ and SGZ neuronal precursors. In the SGZ, VEGF receptor type 2 colocalizes with the immature neuronal marker doublecortin, suggesting a direct action of VEGF on neuronal progenitors (Jin et al. 2002; s. also Sun et al. 2003; Zhu et al. 2003). Consistently, neurogenesis could be inhibited by expression of a dominant negative mutant of this VEGF receptor (Cao et al. 2004).

As mentioned above, recent studies (Davidoff et al. 2004) provided for the first time direct evidence that Leydig cells of the adult rat testis originate from stem-cell-like progenitors that are vascular smooth muscle cells and pericytes of the testicular microvasculature. In this regard, it is important to note that both fetal-like and adult-type Leydig cells arise at the same time, but differ in proliferation and differentiation velocity.

7.8
Leydig Cells May Be Continuously Generated from Stem/Progenitors Cells in the Testes of Adult Mammals

The behaviour and fate of the nestin-positive cells in mature animals represents an interesting item. As established by Davidoff et al. (2004), nestin immunoreactivity was only detectable in the vascular progenitors of the Leydig cells during the formation of the adult-type Leydig cells. In adult rats, after postnatal day 60, nestin immunoreactivity was present not only in periendothelial cells and pericytes of the walls of the microvasculature but also in cells close to these vessels and in certain Leydig cells of the Leydig cell nodules. A similar pattern was observed in testes of adult mice and humans. Thus, it seems likely that during adulthood a low quantity of Leydig cells is continuously produced by transdifferentiation of Leydig stem/progenitor cells. This probably serves to replace old or damaged Leydig cells as well as Leydig cells with impaired functional activity. Such a production of Leydig cells by transdifferentiation of stem/progenitor cells may be also responsible for Leydig cell accumulations during some stages of spermatogenesis known to correlate with local Leydig cell number increases (Bergh 1982, 1983; Paniagua et al. 1988), as well as under conditions leading to Leydig cell hyperplasia in men. That newly formed Leydig cells represent postmitotic cells, generated by transformation of stem/progenitor cells, may explain studies where an increased number but no concomitant division of adult Leydig cells was observed (Ariyaratne and Mendis-Handagama 2000; Ariyaratne et al. 2000a, b, 2003). A continuous production of Leydig cells in adulthood, leading to Leydig cells of variable differentiation stages, may also contribute to the heterogeneity of adult Leydig cell populations.

As itemized in the following, eight important conclusions could be drawn from a recent investigation (Davidoff et al. 2004):

1. The adult stem-cell-like progenitors of the Leydig cells are pericytes and smooth muscle cells of the testis microvasculature.
2. The stem-cell-like progenitors of the testis show nestin, αSMA, NG2, FGF2, PDGFR-ß, and GDNF immunoreactivity and resemble embryonal and adult CNS stem cells.
3. Pericytes become activated and proliferate within 7 days after EDS administration. Daughter cells of these pericytes migrate out from the capillary wall after interrupting the basal lamina and become situated perivascularly as a pool of Leydig cell progenitors.
4. Approximately on day 14 after EDS application, the pericytes in the rat testes start a fast process of transdifferentiation into young (progenitor) Leydig cells (blast-like cells, in analogy to the young neurons or neuroblasts of the nervous system) which acquire steroidogenic and neuroendocrine properties.
5. Newly produced young Leydig cells can undergo a few additional divisions (until the Leydig cell population is completely replenished).
6. A characteristic Leydig cell phenotype emerges rapidly during the transdifferentiation of the pericytes into young Leydig cells, while the pericyte descendants rapidly lose their primordial gene expression pattern. Thus, the stem/progenitor cells of the Leydig cells and their progeny are phenotypically distinguished.
7. All known Leydig cell variants, e.g. precursor-type, progenitor-type, fetal-type, intermediate-type and adult-type Leydig cells, originate from a common ancestor (pericyte/smooth muscle cell) and acquire neuronal, glial and steroidogenic properties. The phenotypic variability of Leydig cells is governed by local environmental factors at the sites where Leydig cells differentiate and function.
8. In adult rat and human testes, new Leydig cells are continuously generated by transdifferentiation of stem-cell-like progenitors. An enhanced transformation of stem-cell-like progenitors into adult-type Leydig cells may result in Leydig cell hyperplasia in men.

As revealed by EDS-induced depletion/regeneration of Leydig cells in the rat (Davidoff et al. 2004), the Leydig cell stem/progenitor cells undergo an initial phase of proliferation (as established by BrdU incorporation) and subsequently transdifferentiate into steroidogenic Leydig cells which rapidly acquire neuronal and glial cell properties. Mainly two Leydig cell phenotypes could be distinguished during the regeneration process in EDS-treated rats: a fetal-type and an adult-type. They arise concomitantly but under distinct environmental and instructive influences and show temporal, spatial, structural and functional differences. Apparently this also holds for Leydig cell formation during normal development in rat and human

(Davidoff et al. 2004), although a different mechanism was proposed elsewhere (Ge et al. 1996). Ge et al. (2005) provided evidence for substantial and stage-dependent changes in the expression of a large number of genes in rat Leydig cells during phased transitions at postnatal days 14-21, 35 and 90. This would be consistent with different waves of Leydig cell generation by transdifferentiation from quiescent pools of stem/progenitor cells (vascular smooth muscle cells and pericytes) in adult rats and humans (Davidoff et al. 2004). Especially in testes of elderly men, numerous newly formed nestin-positive Leydig cells could be seen within areas of Leydig cell hyperplasia. In this respect, transdifferentiation of stem-cell-like progenitors provides a reasonable explanation for the hitherto unresolved question of how increases in Leydig cell number (under conditions of hyperplasia) can occur in the apparent absence of Leydig cell mitotic activity (Davidoff et al. 2004).

7.9
Postnatal Development of Leydig Cells in Rodent Testis

Two distinct Leydig cell phenotypes were described during ontogeny in rodents, viz. fetal-type ones arising during fetal life and adult types occurring at puberty (Dupont et al. 1993; Benton et al. 1995; Haidar 2004). Similarly, both cell types appeared during Leydig cell regeneration following EDS treatment in adult rats. There is evidence for a codistribution and close morphological and functional similarity between the fetal-type Leydig cells remaining after birth and the fetal-like cells arising during postnatal development (Molenaar et al. 1985; Russell et al. 1995). Resulting from the augmentation of total Leydig cell number at days 21-22 after EDS treatment, more testosterone is produced, and the hypertrophic fetal-type Leydig cells become smaller in size, presumably as a result of their adaptation to increasing testosterone delivery by the adult-type Leydig cells. Until the first appearance of the adult-type Leydig cells during postnatal development, the fetal-like Leydig cells alone have to produce those amounts of testosterone necessary for male morphofunctional regulation processes. This may explain why fetal-like Leydig cells appear overstimulated and enlarged. After that, in response to accumulation of testosterone by an additional Leydig cell population, testosterone synthesis per individual cell is reduced, providing a rationale for the phenomenon that the postnatal representatives of the Leydig cell lineage become smaller in size than the fetal ones.

The time of origin of the postnatal Leydig cells has not been exactly determined. Mendis-Handagama et al. (1987) found the first postnatal Leydig cells on day 10 postpartum, whereas Haider et al. (1995) reported the first appearance on postnatal day 13. On the other hand, it has been shown that interstitial stem Leydig cells in a peritubular position become committed to the Leydig cell lineage on day 11 and transform into spindle shaped peritubular Leydig progenitor cells on day 12 (Ariyaratne et al. 2000a; Habert et al. 2001; Zhang et al. 2008). Furthermore, Teerds and Rijntjes (2007) emphasized that the first morphologically recognizable and

3ß-hydroxysteroid dehydrogenase (3ß-HSD)-positive Leydig cells during normal development could be seen between days 7 and 14 postpartum. Moreover, Teerds et al. (2007) reported that spindle-shaped stem Leydig cells of mesenchymal origin, expressing PDGFR-α, the leukaemia inhibitory factor receptor and c-kit but no steroidogenic enzymes and luteinizing hormone (LH) receptors, are the stem cells of the Leydig cells (Ge et al. 2006; Zhang et al. 2008). These cells differentiate into 3ß-HSD-expressing progenitor Leydig cells between postnatal days 10 and 13 and start to proliferate and differentiate between postnatal days 28 and 35 towards immature adult-type Leydig cells. These immature Leydig cells differentiate into mature adult-type Leydig cells from day 56. However, recent investigations on postnatal development of Wistar rats (Davidoff et al. 2004; unpublished observations), using immunohistochemical examinations of nestin (to detect the activated stem cells during processes of proliferation and transdifferentiation towards progenitor Leydig cells) and CytP450scc (to visualize the daughter cells which became Leydig progenitor cells), provided evidence that nestin immunoreactivity in the rat testis can be observed at postnatal day 5 in smooth muscle cells and especially in pericytes within the wall of small blood vessels. In addition, some fetal-type Leydig cell groups in the interstitium were nestin-positive. In the vicinity of these vessels, CytP450scc immunoreactive fetal-type Leydig cell clusters and spindle-shaped cells were seen to contact blood vessel walls located in the vicinity of the seminiferous tubules. These results show that postnatal Leydig cells arise during the first postnatal days and, at postnatal day 5, both intertubular and peritubular stem cells as well as CytP450scc-positive Leydig progenitor cells of two types (clusters of fetal-type cells in the intertubular space and individual spindle-shaped cells with peritubular localization and in contact with small blood vessels) could be observed. At this time, the intertubular clusters (fetal-type Leydig cells) showed a more advanced developmental state (larger size and stronger immunoreactivity for CytP450scc) in comparison with the single spindle-shaped progenitors in peritubular position. From postnatal days 15-28, the number of nestin-positive Leydig stem cells and CytP450scc-positive progenitor Leydig cells with peritubular localization increased. During further development (until postnatal day 60), the fetal-type Leydig cells became smaller, and it was exceedingly difficult to discriminate them from the immature Leydig cells, which predominate between postnatal days 28 and 56 (Zhang et al. 2008). Mature-adult Leydig cells emerge by further differentiation of the immature Leydig cells, which undergo final divisions by day 56 (Hardy et al. 1989; Ge and Hardy 2007). These results provided evidence for a time point characterized by the common presence of both prenatal fetal Leydig cells and postnatally generated fetal-type Leydig cells. Interestingly, on postnatal day 90, a new wave of nestin expression appeared in the vessel walls at intertubular and peritubular positions (Davidoff et al. 2004). The new burst of nestin expression in the adult rat testis points to a process of additional generation of Leydig cells and testosterone production at this developmental period, connected with further maturation of the testis (Haider et al. 1988; Benton et al. 1995; Ariyaratne and Mendis-Handagama 2000).

On the basis of structural and functional criteria, the Leydig progenitor cells resemble mesenchymal stem cells (Ge et al. 1996), detectable in the rat testis between days 14 and 28 postpartum (Hardy et al. 1989; Ge and Hardy 2007). From these, the Leydig progenitor cells are distinguished by the expression of steroidogenic enzymes and LH receptors. Then, the progenitors differentiate further and transform into immature-adult Leydig cells that could be observed between days 28 and 56 postpartum. From day 56 on, the immature Leydig cells develop into adult, highly differentiated Leydig cells with a strongly reduced capability of proliferation (Russell 1996; Teerds 1996; Vergouwen et al. 1991; O'Shaughnessy et al. 2008b). The process of postnatal Leydig cell differentiation has been intensely studied on the basis of morphological features, in particular by examining gene expression of LH and androgen receptors, as well as enzymes involved in steroidogenesis such Cyp11a1 (encodes CytP450scc), cytochrome P450 17α1 (Cyp17A1), 3ß-HSD type1 (Hsd3b1), and 17ß-hydroxysteroid dehydrogenase type 3 (Hsd17b3) (Ge et al. 1996; Shan et al. 1995; Ge and Hardy 2007; O'Shaughnessy et al. 2008b). It was shown that LH and other factors are necessary for the proliferation and differentiation of Leydig cell progenitors (Teerds 1996), and that androgens are required for the differentiation of Leydig cell progenitors into immature Leydig cells (Shan et al. 1995). This is related to the fact that Leydig cell progenitors possess only a few LH receptors but many androgen receptors (Shan and Hardy 1992). It was also established that the human chorionic gonadotropin stimulated conversion of cultured rat Leydig precursor cells to immature Leydig cells is associated with a progressive increase in 5α-reductase activity, which converts the testosterone produced into 5α-reduced metabolites (Murono et al. 1992). Thus, immature Leydig cells actively synthesize but do not secrete testosterone. Testosterone levels increase after postnatal day 40 as a result of progressive decreases in 5α-reductase activity.

According to Ge et al. (1996) and Ge and Hardy (2007), it seems likely that in the adult testis a small population of immature Leydig cells (Leydig cell progenitors) coexists with adult-type Leydig cells. It is believed that under some circumstances these immature (progenitor) Leydig cells serve as a reserve pool for generation of adult Leydig cells in the rat as well as for the permanent replacement of degenerating Leydig cells. Teerds and Rijntjes (2007) reported that only very high doses of human chorionic gonadotropin lead to stimulation of the proliferation ability of a probably existing resting population of Leydig progenitor cells in the adult testis and that some of the Leydig progenitor cells do not reach terminal differentiation and remain in the adult testis as a reserve pool for replacement of destroyed Leydig cells. However, Lauke et al. (1989) have shown that mature human Leydig cells can proliferate in adult human testes bearing early germ cell tumours. It is possible that tumour cell factors secreted into the interstitium of the testis are able to stimulate (reactivate) the proliferative potency of the Leydig cells. Teerds and Rijntjes (2007) proposed local factors which keep the adult Leydig cells in the G0 stage. In this regard, it is of interest to note that the terminally differentiated adult Leydig cells resemble to a certain degree their early progenitor cells, since they retain endocrine, neuroendocrine and mesenchymal stem-cell-like characteristics (Davidoff et al. 2004). In healthy adult human testes as well as in those from patients with Leydig cell hyperplasia, no Leydig cell mitoses could be observed (Davidoff et al. 2004). These results strongly suggest that in the adult testis new Leydig cells arise by transdifferentiation of Leydig stem/progenitor cells which differentiate towards mature Leydig cells.

As discussed above, a lot of neuronal and glial markers become detectable in the Leydig cell progenitors subsequent to the expression of nestin and parallel to the expression of steroidogenic enzymes and LH receptors. Thus, immediately after their appearance, the Leydig cell progenitors acquire neuroendocrine characteristics which remain until adulthood. Recently, an increase in neurofilament heavy polypeptide (Nefh) expression in the progenitor Leydig cells of EDS-treated germ cell-free rats was shown by O'Shaughnessy et al. (2008 b).

7.10
Postnatal Development of Leydig Cells in the Human Testis

According to some authors (Pelliniemi et al. 1996; Huhtaniemi and Pelliniemi 1992; Holstein et al. 1971) the human fetal Leydig cells undergo continuous changes. These include (1) a differentiation phase during fetal weeks 8-14, (2) a fetal maturation phase between weeks 14 and 18 and (3) an involution phase extending from weeks 18 to 38. Mature fetal Leydig cells show specific structural and functional features and form a steroidogenic gland important for the masculinization of the fetus (Pelliniemi et al. 1996). In contrast to previous findings, recent electron-microscopic studies established that cells exhibiting features of steroidogenic activity (smooth endoplasmic reticulum, tubular mitochondria) can be recognized early in the human embryo, namely between the sixth and the seventh postovulatory week, and cells between the seventh and the eighth week show morphological signs of Leydig cells (Makabe et al. 1995).

The postnatal human Leydig cell development follows three stages: a neonatal, an infantile (prepubertal) and a pubertal period (Chemes 1996; Prince 2001). The neonatal period comprises the first two to four postnatal months and is characterized by numerous fetal-type Leydig cells. In this period, the Leydig cells progressively increase in number and reach a maximum at the third postnatal month. Between postnatal months 4 and 12, the Leydig cells rapidly regress, and a heterogeneous population of infantile Leydig cells, myofibroblasts and immature fibroblasts remains in the intertubular space. According to Chemes et al. (1992), the human mesenchymal Leydig cell precursors are capable of producing testosterone. The second period extends between the first year of age and the recognition of the first pubertal signs. During this period, a Leydig cell population exists which resembles dedifferentiated fetal Leydig cells and probably arises from fetal Leydig cells or de novo from Leydig precursor cells. The appearance of the first pubertal signs marks the onset of the third (pubertal) period that extends until sexual maturity is acquired. Fibroblast-like cells proliferate and develop progressively into young and mature Leydig cells. The primary sites of origin of mature Leydig cells are the outer layers of the tubular wall from which these cells migrate towards the intertubular space (Chemes et al. 1992; Chemes 1996; Haider 2004).

Chapter 8
Fetal and Adult Leydig Cells Are of Common Origin

In the developing testis, fetal Leydig cells appear in mice at embryonic day 12.5, in rats at embryonic day 14.5, and in human at weeks 7–8 of pregnancy (Huhtaniemi and Pelliniemi 1992; Pelliniemi et al. 1996; Majdic et al. 1998; Yao and Barsoum 2007). The fetal Leydig cells form clusters that are surrounded by a basal lamina that becomes discontinuous after birth (Kuopio and Pelliniemi 1989; Kuopio et al. 1989a). According to O'Shaugnessy et al. (2006) and Yao and Barsoum (2007), the first visible Leydig cells could be recognized by staining for 3β-hydroxysteroid dehydrogenase or cytochrome P450 side chain cleavage enzyme (CytP450scc) at 12.5 days post coitus (dpc). This occurs after the formation of the testicular cords and the coelomic vessel. At this time, it is not clear whether the first Leydig cells transdifferentiate directly from their stem/progenitors within the gonadal mesenchyme or via stem/progenitor Leydig cells (pericytes) in the testicular vasculature. After initial differentiation and proliferation of fetal Leydig cells around day 12 of gestation (Gondos 1980), the fetal Leydig cell population remains virtually unchanged in mice, and, for example, the number of Leydig cells is stable between day 16 of gestation and day 5 after birth (Baker and O'Shaughnessy 2001a). This suggests that the fetal Leydig cells are terminally differentiated and do not divide (Zhang et al. 2008). However, there are also reports indicating that the number of fetal Leydig cells increases between embryonic days 17 and 21 or immediately before birth (Kerr et al. 1988). The latter would not be compatible with the idea that fetal Leydig cells arise by transdifferentiation from stem/progenitor Leydig cells in analogy with the adult Leydig cell population. After birth, the number of fetal Leydig cells significantly decreases. In contrast, Kerr and Knell (1988) proposed that 50–75% of the original "fetal-type" Leydig cell population present at birth persists in the adult testis. In this context, observations (Davidoff et al. 2004) that "fetal-type" Leydig cells are generated during postnatal development are significant, since these cells could be hardly distinguished from the prenatal fetal Leydig cells.

During prenatal testis development in rats and mice, nestin immunoreactivity was found to be temporally expressed in Sertoli cells as well as in myofibroblasts and other undefined cells of the interstitium (Fröjdman et al. 1997). At 12 dpc, nestin immunoreactivity was detectable in cells of mesonephric mesenchyme surrounding the mesonephric tubules and in cells below the surface epithelium. At 13 dpc, strong immunoreactivity was established in cells of the gonadal blastema below the surface epithelium. A characteristic localization was the basal cytoplasm of Sertoli cells. Cells of the interstitium showed moderate staining intensity, whereas the prospective myofibroblasts of the lamina propria were strongly marked. Until birth, this staining pattern did not change significantly.

Concerning the not yet identified origin of the fetal Leydig cells, Yao and Barsoum (2007) recently discussed multiple potential sources, in particular the adrenal-gonadal primordium, neural crest, mesonephros and coelomic epithelium (Karl and Capel 1998; Brennan et al. 2003; Buher et al. 1993; Merchant-Larios and Moreno-Mendoza 1998; Nishino et al. 2001; O'Shaughnessy et al. 2006). As indicated within this review, there are considerable arguments for a neuroectodermal, neural crest origin of these cells, which may reach the male gonad by migration from the mesonephros stromal network into the gonad anlage and as a component of the coelomic vessel of the XY gonad (cf. Coveney et al. 2008; Cool et al. 2008; see later).

8.1
Where Do the Leydig Cell Ancestors Come from?

Studies on the development of the rat and human Leydig cells gave no direct answer to this question, because early neuroectodermal cells seem to migrate towards their final destination (organ) in the form of spindle-shaped cells (Frésen et al. 1995), morphologically resembling embryonic mesenchymal cells or cells of the loose connective tissue. In addition, during this migration, the mesenchymal-like Leydig cells cease the expression of their specific marker substances (Ge et al. 2005, 2006; Hardy and Ge 2007; Zhang et al. 2008). This is the reason why most of the investigators who worked on this topic speculated that the Leydig cell progenitors must be cells of mesenchymal origin and shape, and focused their observations and main interest on the cells of the mesenchyme (Hardy et al. 1989; Teerds 1996; Teerds et al. 1999; Ariyaratne et al. 2000 a, b; Ge et al. 2006).

The place of origin of the stem-cell-like progenitors of Leydig cells is still unknown. There is evidence that neuroectodermal derivatives may derive from the neural tube, the neural crest (Dahlstrand et al. 1995) and neuroectodermal placodes or from the entire surface neuroectoderm. Moreover, endodermal derivatives may also originate from the neural plate during gastrulation. Thus, the strict separation of the main embryological layers (ectoderm, mesoderm and endoderm) has to be revised. The mesenchyme, which represents the embryonic connective tissue, is a mix of cells originating from the main embryological layers (Chemes 1996; Ge et al. 1996).

Where do the stem-cell-like progenitors move through to arrive at their final destination? There are various possibilities, such as migration through the mesoderm or mesenchyme (mesectoderm, ectomesoderm, including the mesonephros), along with epithelial cells of tubular organs as in the pancreas (endomesoderm) or as shown by Davidoff et al. (2004) along growing blood vessels during angiogenesis, representing a structural component of their wall (Coveney et al. 2008). Fröjdman et al. (1997) provided evidence for nestin immunoreactivity at 13 dpc in cells of the testis interstitium. In addition, it was established that the vessels recognized in the rat testis parenchyma at days 19–20 of fetal life contained nestin-immunoreactive cells in their thin walls (Davidoff, unpublished). Thus, the association of stem-cell-like progenitors and blood vessels occurs early in the embryogenesis of the testis (cf. Brennan and Capel 2004).

8.2
The Development of the Fetal Leydig Cells Is Closely Associated with the Development of the Testis Vasculature

As mentioned already, the vascular wall is a source of stem cells (Tavian et al. 2005). The morphology and functional features of testicular vasculature have been described repeatedly (Setchell et al. 1994; Sharpe 1994).

Weerasooriya and Yamamoto (1985) studied the structure of muscular venules in the interstitial columns and established, by cross-sections, the casts of the testicular microvessels showing a characteristic hexagonal pattern; usually there is one intertubular vessel (an arteriole, a capillary or a venule) per intertubular column, and one layer of loosely spaced peritubular vessels between two neighbouring seminiferous tubules. The intertubular and peritubular capillaries join to form intertubular or peritubular venules and muscular venules which are commonly located in interstitial columns. The venous branches thereafter seem to run in a centrifugal manner towards the surface forming the outermost layer of testicular vasculature. The outermost vascular layer consists of veins, venules and capillaries; arterial elements are not encountered, and there is only one subalbugineal venous plexus.

One of the earliest features of gonadal differentiation is the divergent pattern of the vasculature in XX and XY gonads (Brennan et al. 2002; Brennan and Capel 2004; Yao et al. 2006). Between 11.5 and 12.5 dpc a large vessel on the coelomic surface of the XY gonad, the coelomic vessel, could be observed. This is a specific artery which seems to be critical for testis development and hormone transport. The formation of the coelomic vessel neither requires Sertoli cell differentiation nor Sry (Yao et al. 2004), but requires inhibin β B (which contributes to its proper formation). Indeed, testis-determining genes of the XY gonad, including Sry and/or Sox9 (Kobayashi et al. 2005), are thought to suppress Wnt4 expression, allowing activin B to work with other factors, such as transforming growth factor β proteins, to facilitate coelomic vessel formation. It seems very likely that the cellular components of this coelomic vessel represent migrating cells of the mesonephros. Recent findings by Coveney et al. (2008) confirm this presumption. These authors, using time-lapse microscopy, described the origin of the XY-specific coelomic vessel in cultured mice gonads in detail. They found that at 11.5 dpc a large blood vessel plexus is present in the mesonephros and small vascular branches extend across the gonad boundary. During the first steps of differentiation of the testis (characterized by the expression of Sry), at 12.0 dpc the vascular plexus in the mesonephros dissolved, and the individual endothelial cells released migrated along restricted tracks towards the specified coelomic epithelial domain and between regions where testis cords were assembling, and at 12.5 dpc cells generated the specific coelomic vessel and its branches.

The endothelial cells of newly generated endothelial tubes recruit pericyte progenitors that contribute to the stabilization of the new blood vessels. Coveney et al. (2008) did not study this phase of the generation of the testicular vasculature. However, it can be presumed that pericyte precursors migrate together with endothelial cells from the mesonephros into the developing gonad (Brennan and Capel 2004). An alternative possibility is that the pericyte progenitors preexist in the aorta–gonad–mesonephros (AGM) region as stromal cells which are recruited during the assembly of the male-specific coelomic vessel (Majesky 2007). Alternatively, pericytes could be produced by migrating endothelial cells themselves (Cossu and Bianco 2003).

The results obtained by Cui et al. (2004) provide further evidence for the close relationship between Leydig cells and the vascular muscle cells/pericyte lineage. These authors were able to show in Pod1 (capsulin/epicardin/Tcf21) knockout male mice the absence of the characteristic coelomic vessel associated with pericyte disturbances and markedly decreased endothelial cell migration from mesonephros. In control animals, Pod1 was expressed in the indifferent gonad at 11.5 dpc, subsequently localizing to the interstitial region of the developing testis. By 18.5 dpc, the Pod1-directed LacZ reporter in the testes was expressed in peritubular myofibroblasts, fetal Leydig cells and pericytes surrounding blood vessels. Therefore, Cui et al. (2004) proposed that expansion of the Leydig cell population is associated with the loss of the peritubular myoid cells and pericytes, which under these experimental conditions leads to disruption of the organization of testicular structure and vasculature (Cui et al. 2003).

8.3
Leydig Cells, Blood Vessels and the Developing Testis

A narrow relationship between the emergence of Leydig cells and testicular vasculature also appears to exist during early development of the male mouse gonad (Brennan et al. 2002, 2003; Yao et al. 2002; Jeays-Ward et al. 2003). The gonad appears as a thickening along the ventromedial side of the mesonephros at approximately 10.5 dpc. First, the structure of this gonad anlage is identical in XX and XY mice embryos. At 10.5 dpc in XY embryos, expression of Sry by pre-Sertoli cells is initiated (Koopman et al. 1990, 1991; Lovell-Badge and Robertson 1990), resulting in proliferation of the coelomic epithelium (Schmahl et al. 2000), cell migration from mesonephros into the gonad and testis cord formation (Buher et al. 1993; Merchnat-Larios et al. 1993; Martineau et al. 1997; Capel et al. 1999; Schmahl et al. 2000; Brennan et al. 2002, 2003). At 11.5 dpc, upregulation of Sox9 is established. This leads to massive migration of mesonephric cells, which develop into peritubular myoid, endothelial and myoepithelial (perivascular) cells (Buehr et al. 1993; Martineau et al. 1997; Tilmann and Capel 1999; Brennan et al. 2002). However, a recent study by Cool et al. (2008), using enhanced yellow fluorescent protein (EYFP)–α-smooth muscle actin (αSMA) transgenic mice, showed no migration of αSMA-EYFP-positive cells from the mesonephros during the period when migration is required for testis cord formation. The only cells migrating from the mesonephros were endothelial cells. These cells contributed, between 11.5 and 12.5 dpc, to the formation of the coelomic vessel. The same mesonephric migrating cells contribute to the branches of the coelomic vessel, which are subsequently visible and directed towards the interstitial space of the testis lying in the vicinity of developing testicular cords. These events coincide with the generation of the first haematopoietic stem cells (HSCs) in the dorsal aorta and mesenchyme at embryonic day 11.0 as well as in the urogenital ridges at embryonic day 12.0. During this period, the AGM region and especially the urogenital ridge subregion yielded more supportive clones for HSCs than adult bone marrow stromal cells (Oostendorp et al. 2002). In addition, there is evidence that most HSC-supportive lines are midway between a true mesenchymal phenotype and a fully differentiated vascular smooth muscle phenotype (Remy-Martin et al. 1999).

The use of different experimental approaches leads to the interesting conclusion that the Leydig cell progenitors are already present in the gonad by day 11.5 and are not derived from the mesonephros after this stage (Yao et al. 2002; Jeays-Ward et al. 2003). In addition, labelling experiments, performed by Brennan et al. (2003), showed that the coelomic epithelium during the SF-1-proliferative stage is not a major source for the Leydig cell lineage. Differentiated Leydig cells were seen at 12.5 dpc following the development of testis cords and the male-specific vasculature. Leydig cell differentiation requires Desert hedgehog, which is produced by Sertoli cells (Clark et al. 2000; Yao et al. 2002; Park et al. 2007). Treatment with forskolin completely inhibits mesonephric cell migration and Leydig cell differentiation. In this case, the appearance of Leydig cells in the absence of mesonephric cell migration indicates that either Leydig cells derive from other sources, such as the coelomic epithelium of the gonad (Karl and Capel 1998) or Leydig cell precursors migrate into the gonad before 11.5 dpc as a component of a non-committed stem/progenitor cell population (Yao et al. 2002; Tilman and Capel 2002; Brennan et al. 2002, 2003). In addition, these studies show that Leydig cell progenitors represent a stable cell population which cannot be damaged easily. In accordance, the results obtained by Davidoff et al. (2004) show that ethane dimethanesulphonate administration in adult rats destroys the existing adult Leydig cell population, but not their stem-cell-like progenitors, which retain their capability to produce a new population of Leydig cells (Teerds et al. 1999; Aryiaratne et al. 2003). In accordance with this cells and pericytes, studies on platelet derived growth factor (PDGF) A, PDGF receptor α (PDGFR-α), PDGF-B and PDGF receptor ß (PDGFR-ß) deficient mice showed a lack of development of pericytes in the microvasculature and of alveolar smooth muscle cells in the lung (Lindahl et al. 1997a, b; Hellström et al. 1999, 2001; Lindblom et al. 2003) as well as of severely impaired Leydig cell precursor proliferation, differentiation and migration (Gnessi et al. 2000; Brennan et al. 2003).

As mentioned above, HSCs within the AGM region of the embryonic mouse migrate into the genital ridge concomitantly with other stem cells (e.g. endothelial stem cells, neural crest stem cells, mesenchymal stem cells) (Ohneda et al. 1998; Britsch et al. 1998; Oostendorp et al. 2002). Thus, the gonad anlage receives and possesses an abundant collection of diverse stem cells which are present at 9.5, 10.5 and 11.5 dpc, respectively. This is the time when the gonad appears for the first time as a small thickening of the ventromedial mesonephros. Because a number of stem cells seem to posses the capability to differentiate into neural cells (see above), it can be presumed that some stem cells of the AGM region are incorporated into the coelomic/testicular vessel wall during its assembly as mural cells (smooth muscle cells and pericytes) (Brennan et al. 2002, 2003; Cool et al. 2008). These cells provide the reserve (quiescent) stem cell pool, from which Leydig cells emerge after appropriate local environmental signals.

In a recent study, Tang et al. (2008) revealed the importance of the Notch signalling pathway (Lai 2004; Collesi et al. 2008; Campa et al. 2008) for the maintenance of the Leydig cell progenitors in the fetal mouse testis. It is important to note that Notch signalling did not affect committed Leydig cell fate. This study supports our proposal that fetal and adult Leydig cells share the same ancestor. Furthermore, the results obtained by Tang et al. (2008) support our view that the fetal Leydig cell progenitors may be components of the specific testis vasculature, namely the pericytes of the coelomic vessel. In accordance, these authors established that Notch ligands such as Jagged 2, delta-like 1, delta-like 3 and delta-like 4 are expressed at 11.5 and 12.5 dpc in the XY gonad, particularly and specifically in the coelomic vessel and its branches (Brennan et al. 2002; Nef et al. 2005; Sainson and Harris 2008). Representing a further result of significance, only undifferentiated progenitor cells were responsive to active Notch signalling. Tang et al. (2008) hypothesized that mesenchymal Leydig stem/progenitor cells arise in the gonad at early developmental stages and that some of these cells differentiate into fetal Leydig cells during embryonic development, whereas others retain their undifferentiated characteristics and serve as stem cells/precursors of Leydig cells during postnatal testis development. This is compatible with our view that pericytes of the testicular vessel walls are Leydig cell progenitors (Armulik et al. 2005; Scehnet et al. 2007; Jin et al. 2008; Weber 2008; da Silva Meirelles et al. 2008). In this regard, it is important to recollect, that the cardiovascular system is the first organ system that emerges during embryonic development. Thus, the blood vessels derive from (and may still contain) very early stem/progenitor cells (e.g. pericytes). Subsequently organs develop around invading blood vessels (Nikolova and Lammert 2003), and pericytes/smooth muscle cells recruited during angiogenesis can remain as quiescent (silencing) stem/progenitor mural cells. In response to activation by appropriate epigenetic factors, these cells can then act as a source to provide different cell types for organogenesis during embryonic development and for reparation/regeneration processes in damaged adult organs (see Sect. 7.5; Armulik et al. 2005). Endorsing the functional significance of Notch in vascular smooth muscle cells, recent findings revealed that PDGFR-β (PDGF-BB is critically important for vascular development and for the homeostasis of blood vessels) represents a novel Notch immediate downstream gene and is regulated by Notch 1 and Notch 3 signalling (Jin et al. 2008; Weber 2008).

The substantial similarity in the guidance and patterning modes between the nervous system and the vasculature has to be emphasized. During patterning, bidirectional crosstalk between both systems seems to exist, and the same molecular signal pathways were found during guidance in both nervous and vascular systems (see Carmeliet 2003; Carmeliet and Tessier-Lavigne 2005; Weinstein 2005, for reviews). These results further support the possibility that neural cells may develop from vessel components.

To assess the expression levels of nestin during development, we carried out comparative immunoblot analyses in testes of different ontogenetic stages (Davidoff et al. 2004). These studies showed an elevated nestin expression in this organ until postnatal day 15, with the highest levels at day 5 and a new increase at day 90 (Fig. 8.1).

The examination of CytP450scc levels during postnatal development revealed a biphasic protein expression pattern: CytP450scc levels were initially (at day 5) significantly higher than at days 10 and 15 (decreased number of fetal-type Leydig cells), but with the appearance and increase of the number of adult Leydig cells the expression increased thereafter (between days 24 and 27) to attain maximal (e.g. adult) values (Fig. 8.1).

8.4
Are Stem Cells Really a Very Rare Population?

A common feature of stem/progenitor cells in different organs is their very low number (Kuznetsov et al. 2007). This was also observed in the case of the progenitors of the Leydig cells which have characteristics similar to those of other types of stem cells such as HSCs (Lo et al. 2004; Ge et al. 2006, 2007). Pericytes do not exist as free cells within testicular interstitium (mesenchyme), but are surrounded by the basement membrane of the microvasculature within their specific vascular niches. They may not have been released under previous conditions applied for isolation of the mesenchymal stem cells, presumed to be Leydig stem cells (Ge et al. 2006; Teerds et al. 2007). Pericyte isolation requires particular experimental conditions (Péault et al. 2007). Pericytes do not express steroidogenic enzymes and luteinizing hormone receptors, characteristic for their progeny, the Leydig cells. This enabled the immunohistochemical examination of the transdifferentiation process. After ceasing their proliferative activity, the pericytes remain in the vascular niches as a quiescent (resting) reserve pool of stem/progenitor cells for future physiological repair and regeneration of Leydig cells (Young 2004).

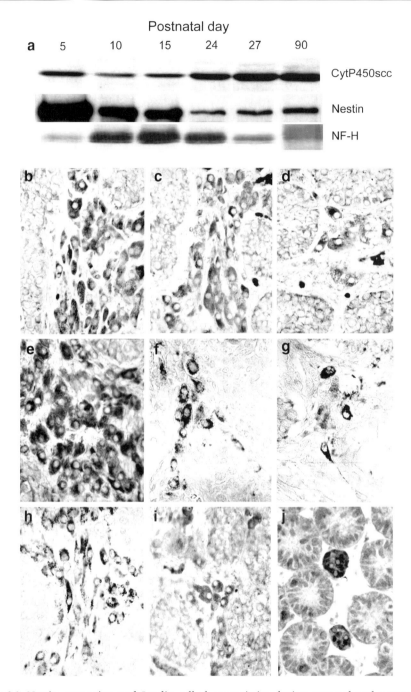

Fig. 8.1 Nestin expression and Leydig cell characteristics during prenatal and postnatal development in the human and rat testis. Immunoblots show striking alterations in cytochrome P450 side chain cleavage enzyme, nestin and neurofilament protein 200 levels

From the consideration that adult stem cells of one organ after transplantation into another organ can differentiate into cells characteristic for the host organ and that adult stem cells can be transported to other organs by the blood circulation, as evident in the case of bone marrow stem cells, such mechanisms were thought to have a general significance for the regeneration of damaged organs. This seems to be also true for the testis, because bone marrow stem cells differentiate in testis not only into Sertoli cells within seminiferous tubules and into Leydig cells in the interstitium (Yazawa et al. 2006), but also into spermatogonia and spermatocytes (Nayernia et al. 2006; Lue et al. 2007; Drusenheimer et al. 2007). On the other hand, isolated spermatogonial stem cells from adult mouse testis may dedifferentiate in culture towards embryonal-like stem cells capable of generating progeny representatives of all three germ layers, including cardiomyocytes (Guan et al. 2007). Recently, Kucia et al. (2007) revealed in bone marrow a population of very small embryonic-like stem cells which were deposited during embryogenesis and are descendants from the epiblast. These cells migrate through the AGM splanchnopleura to the fetal liver and subsequently to the bone marrow. Interestingly, these cells express neural lineage markers and form neurospheres in vitro (Kucia et al. 2006b). Very small embryonic stem cells may also reach other organs and remain there for a certain time period in a quiescent state (Kucia et al. 2006a, d). Recently, da Silva Meirelles et al. (2006, 2008) confirmed that mesenchymal stem cells reside in virtually all postnatal organs and tissues but not in the blood. The distribution of the mesenchymal stem cells throughout the postnatal organism is related to their existence in a perivascular niche. Regarding the observation that most mesenchymal stem cell progenitor types exhibit essential similarity with pericytes and that certain mesenchymal stem cells established in the body represent pericyte descendants (Dellavalle et al. 2007), we propose that mesenchymal stem cells in the perivascular niches of different organs are daughter cells of pericytes (da Silva Meirelles et al. 2008). Hereby, pericytes could be the ancestor cells of all adult stem cells in the organism (cf. Covas et al. 2008).

There is accumulating evidence that diverse organs exhibit their own specific stem cells, which are able to support most effectively repair processes (da Silva Meirelles et al. 2006, 2008), including the side population stem cells of the testis (Kubota et al. 2003; Shimizu et al. 2006; Lo et al. 2004). Moreover, transplantation of foreign stem cells into a host organ does not contribute essentially to repair and regeneration processes (Coyne et al. 2006), and no mesenchymal stem cells were

Fig. 8.1 (continued) during rat testis postnatal development. Immunohistochemical analyses on human testis sections demonstrate Leydig-cell-associated immunoreactivity for TrkA at the 18th (b), 25th (c) and 33rd (d) weeks of gestation, for tyrosine hydroxylase at the 16th (e), 29th (f) and 34th (g) weeks of gestation as well as for glial cell line derived neurotrophic factor at the 16th (h) and 30th (i) weeks of gestation. Note the decreases in Leydig cell number and staining intensity during ontogeny. j Rat Leydig cells at postnatal day 5 show abundant vascular endothelial growth factor immunoreactivity (a–i ×250; j ×230). (Data in a derived from Davidoff et al. 2004)

found in the blood (da Silva Meirelles et al. 2006). While transplantation of muscle pericytes into the skeletal musculature generated limited activity concerning muscle repair or regeneration (Dellavale et al. 2007), muscle pericytes injected into the bloodstream showed substantial reparation/regeneration ability (Péault et al. 2007) by stimulating the intrinsic pericyte population and it progeny, namely the satellite cells of skeletal muscle (Peng and Huard 2004). Thus, the true stem/progenitors of these organs might be the microvascular pericytes (Covas et al. 2008).

8.5
Leydig Stem/Progenitor Cells and the Neural Crest

8.5.1
Are Pericytes and Leydig Cells of Neuroectodermal/Neural Crest Origin?

The stem-cell-like progenitors of Leydig cells possess striking similarities with stem/progenitor cells of the developing or adult central and peripheral nervous system and especially with cells of the neural crest in relation to their nestin, αSMA, vascular endothelial growth factor, basic fibroblast growth factor and endothelial growth factor receptor immunoreactivity. Neural crest stem cells are located at the border of the neural plate ectoderm and the non-neural ectoderm. Neural crest cells arise after an epitheliomesenchymal transdifferentiation (Pla et al. 2001; Pla and Larue 2003; Trainor et al. 2003). Neural stem cells and neural crest stem cells are able to differentiate into smooth muscle cells (Galli et al. 2000; Rietze et al. 2001; Oishi et al. 2002). Recently, Pierret et al. (2006) proposed that peripheral, tissue-derived, or adult stem cells (including those from bone marrow and blood vessels) are all progeny of the neural crest.

In 1987, after establishing expression of substance P and methionine-enkephalin in human Leydig cells, Schulze et al. (1987a) asked whether these cells are of neural (neural crest) origin. Subsequently, substance P immunoreactivity, messenger RNA and protein as well a second neural marker, neuron-specific enolase, were established in Leydig cells of other species (Chivakata et al. 1991; Angelova and Davidoff 1991; Angelova et al. 1991a–c). That Leydig cells express neural markers was confirmed by Mayerhofer et al. (1992, 1996), who demonstrated that adult mouse, rat and hamster Leydig cells (as well as mesonephros-derived cells that migrate into testis during development) express the neural cell adhesion molecule. Through the application of immunohistochemical, western blot, PCR and in situ hybridization techniques, the expression of a large number of neuronal, neuroendocrine and glial marker substances by Leydig cells of human and rodent testes has been demonstrated (see Chap. 3; Davidoff et al. 1993, 1996, 2002; Middendorff et al. 1993; Müller et al. 2006). On the basis of these results, it has been concluded that Leydig cells are distinguished by both mesodermal and neuroendocrine properties and they were defined as a member of the diffuse neuroendocrine system. According to these features, Leydig cells resemble neural crest cells.

It is well known that during development of the nervous system, the early nestin expression by neural stem cells is replaced by other intermediate filament proteins, namely neurofilament proteins in neurons and glial fibrillary acidic protein (GFAP) in glial cells (Dahlstrand et al. 1995; Doetsch et al. 1999a, b; Alvarez-Buylla et al. 2001, 2002; Doetsch 2003a). In 2004, Davidoff et al. showed that the Leydig cell progenitors and the newly formed Leydig cells behave as neural cell progenitors initially expressing nestin and in a later phase neural and glial cell proteins. They also found that the high molecular weight proteoglycan NG2, which is expressed by oligodendrocyte progenitors as well as by smooth muscle cells and pericytes during vascular morphogenesis, exhibits a similar developmental pattern during postnatal generation of the Leydig cells (Belachew et al. 2003; Ozerdem et al. 2001). The fact that nestin is also temporally expressed by muscle cells during early embryonal development could be explained by the existence of two enhancer elements in the first and the second intron of the nestin gene which are responsible for nestin expression in muscle and nerve cells, respectively (Zimmerman et al. 1994; Josephson et al. 1998). These results show that nestin expression is not absolutely specific for nerve cell progenitors. However, the combination of nestin expression together with the expression of further genes and products, characteristic for the neural cell lineage, permit the conclusion that Leydig cell progenitors possess true neural progeny. This can explain their rapid transformation and differentiation towards the neuroendocrine cell lineage. The fact that newly formed Leydig cells, soon after emergence, rapidly lose their proliferation capacity explains their unusual terminal differentiation to a multipotent, postmitotic cell type which comprises steroidogenic, neural and glial cell characteristics.

It is of interest that Leydig cells do not represent the only cell type with neural properties that is capable of synthesizing steroid hormones. Neurons as well as central and peripheral glial cells are also able to produce steroid hormone metabolites (Davidoff et al. 2002). Moreover, it is not surprising that Leydig cells possess glial markers. It is well known that neural stem cells may differentiate into neurons and glial cells. Recent data showed that radial glial cells may also be progenitors of neocortical neurons (Tamamaki et al. 2001). Thus, Leydig cells achieve a terminal differentiation that resembles a multipotent progenitor cell type that has lost its ability to divide. But during the whole of life Leydig cells are continuously substituted by transdifferentiated adult stem/progenitor cells (pericytes, smooth muscle cells).

Extensive work (Schulze et al. 1987; Davidoff et al. 1995; 1996; 2002, 2004, 2005; Middendorff et al. 1993, 1995, 1996, 1997a–c, 2000a, b, 2002; Müller et al. 2006) has revealed that the Leydig cell of vertebrate testes represents a cell type distinguished by a complex phenotype, covering epithelial, mesenchymal, myofibroblastic, endocrine and neuroendocrine characteristics. Most probably, both fetal and adult Leydig cells retain some of the phenotypical properties of their ancestors. As discussed above, the pericytes may derive from neural crest cells or from a common stem cell population segregated early in embryogenesis with progeny for both the neural crest and the mesoderm lineage (mesectoderm, mesenchymal–neural).

As established by Le Douarin et al. (2004, 2008) in vertebrate embryos, neuroectodermal neural crest cells exhibit a remarkable broad potential, giving rise, after a migratory phase, to neurons and glial cells in the peripheral nervous system and to skin melanocytes, all designated as "neural" derivatives. Neural-crest-derived cells also include non-neural, "mesenchymal" cell types such as chondrocytes and bone cells, myofibroblasts and adipocytes, which largely contribute to the head structures in amniotes (Crane and Trainor 2006; Le Douarin et al. 2007; Billon et al. 2007; Dupin et al. 2007). Similar to findings in the blood cell system, recent findings established the presence of multipotent progenitors endowed with both mesenchymal and neural differentiation capacities in early migratory neural crest cells of the avian embryo. This "mesenchymal–neural" clonogeneic cell type is upstream of all the other neural crest progenitors known so far and shows increased activity in response to Sonic hedgehog (Calloni et al. 2007; Le Douarin et al. 2008). The "mesenchymal–neural" precursor cells (Mujtaba et al. 1998; Le Douarin et al. 2004, 2008; Pouget et al. 2006; Calloni et al. 2007; Müller et al. 2008; Foster et al. 2008), which become integrated into microvascular niches during development and propagation of the vasculature, may be defined as resting (silencing) progenitors. The pericytes behave principally as stem cells because, located in the vascular niches of various organs (Bianco and Cosu 1999; De Angelis et al. 1999; Palmer et al. 2000; Minasi et al. 2002; Lin et al. 2008; Morrison and Spradling 2008), they give rise to a large number of different cell types, including the Leydig cells, after activation. Thus, pericytes of the microvasculature, generally acting as stem/progenitor cells in the body, represent a population of restricted precursor cells in individual organs (nervous system, muscle, skeleton, skin, liver, testis), where they generate intermediate and differentiated adult organ-specific cells (Rao 2004a; Tavian et al. 2005; Ge et al. 2005, 2006; Teerds et al. 2007). Notably, mesenchymal stromal cells derived from the human bone marrow have the potential to differentiate into neuronal cells with specific gene expression and functional properties (Tondreau et al. 2004, 2008). Similarly, cardiac neural-crest-derived cells contribute to the dormant multipotent stem cells which differentiate under appropriate conditions into cardiomyocytes, peripheral nervous system type neurons, glial cells and smooth muscle cells (Tomita et al. 2005). Recently, a new population of very small embryonic-like stem cells characterized by markers of neural-tissue-committed stem cells was isolated from bone marrow and other organs (Ratajczak et al. 2008). These cells, expressing neural lineage markers such as βIII-tubulin, nestin, NeuN, and GFAP, were shown to be able to form neurospheres in vitro and to be mobilized into the peripheral blood following stroke (Kucia et al. 2006b).

Because of the similarities between fetal and adult Leydig cells, both populations may have a common origin. As discussed above, pericyte progenitors or differentiated pericytes represent possible candidate precursors of fetal Leydig cells. Besides the neural crest, pericytes may originate from an earlier stem cell type of neuroectodermal origin, the recently discovered multipotent "mesenchymal–neural" stem cells (Calloni et al. 2007; Le Douarin 2008) or from epiblast (primitive ectoderm) stem cells, designated as "very small embryonic-like stem cells" (Kucia et al. 2006d).

These multipotent mesenchymal–neural stem cells were found to be the precursors of the neural crest and could also act as the ancestor cell type for the pericytes.

8.5.2
Differences Between Neural Crest Cells from Head and Trunk Regions

It is well known that neural crest cells from the head region differ from those of the trunk region concerning their ability to produce mesenchymal progeny (Bergwerff et al. 1998; Le Douarin et al. 2008). Recent results provided evidence that derivatives of trunk neural crest cells (Schwann cells) not only resume developmental pathways specific for their neural crest precursors (melanocytic differentiation), but also can recapitulate a certain mesenchymal potential (myofibroblasts), expressed in vivo by the cephalic neural crest cells (Real et al. 2005, 2006). At postmigratory stages, differentiated neural crest cell derivatives with a remarkable phenotypic plasticity were observed (Dupin et al. 2007). For example, epidermal pigment cells and Schwann cells from peripheral nerves were able in single-cell culture to reattain multipotent neural-crest-like features endowed with self-renewal. Thus, stem cell properties are directed by a variety of neural crest progenitors, and they can be reacquired in differentiated cells from neural crest origin, providing the possibility to act in repair and regeneration processes.

Indicating the ability to provide mesenchymal lineage progeny, Pouget et al. (2006) showed that somites give rise to smooth muscle cells and endothelial cells of the trunk aorta (Wasteson et al. 2008; Ben-Yair and Kalcheim 2008). Pouget et al. (2008) revealed that both vascular smooth muscle cells and pericytes of the trunk aorta originate in the sclerotome of somites (Brand-Saberi and Christ 2000; Christ et al. 2004), whereas pericytes of the viscera were not of somite/sclerotomal origin. Migrating neural crest cells reach the sclerotome during early embryogenesis. This raises the possibility that smooth muscle cells of neural crest origin also allocate the thoracic aorta and probably its branching blood vessels in testis (Moore and Larue 2004). In apparent support, Joseph et al. (2004) established that trunk neural crest cells actually adopt a myofibroblast fate in vivo (see Esner et al. 2006, for the dorsal aorta), suggesting that pericytes invade the endoneurial space along with blood vessels. However, the authors established that nerve pericytes are not neural-crest-derived. In this regard, Howson et al. (2005) have recently shown that the postnatal rat aorta contains an immature subpopulation of anchorage-independent mesenchymal cells with pericyte progenitor features. These cells were termed "spheroid forming aortic cells" (SFACs) on the basis of their capacity to form spheroids in suspension culture. SFACs express CD34 and Tie-2 and test negative for CD31, endothelial-type nitric oxide synthase, Flk-1, and αSMA, a protein repertoire compatible with a primitive, undifferentiated phenotype. These cells also test positive for markers of early pericyte lineage (NG2, nestin, PDGFR-α, PDGFR-β, calponin and desmin). Upon treatment with serum, SFACs lose their capacity to grow in suspension and differentiate into a CD34-negative, αSMA-positive mural cell phenotype while still testing negative for markers of endothelial cell differentiation.

There is also evidence that cells in the dorsal aorta and the myotome have a common clonal origin.

8.5.3
The Potential Neural Crest Origin of the Leydig Cells and the Restricted Experimental Applicability of LacZ Transgenic Mice

Using two types of transgene mice, namely the reporter lines PO=::Cre;R26R (Yamauchi et al. 1999) and Wnt1::Cre;R26R (Chai et al. 2000), which express LacZ (β-galactosidase), Brennan et al. (2003) found no evidence for the contribution of the neural crest to the development of testicular Leydig cells (Yao and Barsoum 2007). Since Leydig cells (and other testicular cells) were shown to possess endogenous LacZ enzyme activity (Davidoff et al. 2004; see Molenaar et al. 1986a), using mice with targeted mutations in genes of the neural-crest-specific neuregulin receptors ErbB2 and ErbB3 (Britsch et al. 1998), a reliable examination of testes from LacZ mice has to be precluded. This problem was recently discussed more broadly for cells from the bone marrow by Kopp et al. (2007). Thus, the possibility that Leydig cells may originate from migrating neural crest cells cannot be rejected by the study cited above (Brennan et al. 2003). However, there also exists the possibility that Leydig cells and neural crest cells have a common ancestor. Such a cell, present in the very early stage of development, should have characteristics of early embryonic-like cells that are able to differentiate into both neural crest cells and pericyte progenitors (see Sect. 8.5.1). Some of these cells could move with the blood vessels which grow into newly formed organs and remain there as quiescent (silence) pluripotent stem cells.

A probable origin of the pericytes in visceral organs and the developing testis is the paraaortic splanchopleura and the AGM region in avian and mammalian (including human) embryos (see Majesky 2007, for a review).

8.6
The Aorta–Gonad–Mesonephros Region Harbours Many Diverse Stem Cells

Although the origin of multipotent HSCs is still controversial, the AGM region (in mouse and human) and the paraaortic splanchnopleura (in chick) are widely accepted as the areas of their origin (Kubo and Alitalo 2003).

The AGM region represents a space of the murine embryonic splanchnopleuric mesoderm, bounded by the dorsal aorta, gonadal ridge and promesoneophros. The AGM region has been identified as a potent source of HSCs at 8.5–10.5 dpc, preceding their appearance in fetal liver.

There is a remarkable similarity between the bone marrow stroma and the mesenchymal region including the paraaortic splanchopleura/AGM regions (Matsuoka et al. 2001; Nadin et al. 2003) in the mouse embryo. In these regions, high expression of the stem cell factor was revealed during embryogenesis, playing an important role in cells associated with migratory pathways and homing sites of melanoblasts, germ cells and HSCs as well as stem cell proliferation, differentiation or survival in late development (Matsui et al. 1990; Keshet et al. 1991; Sieber-Blum and Hu 2008). Both areas contain a large number of different stem/progenitor cells (Herzog et al. 2003; Medvinsky et al. 1993; Godin et al. 1993; Yoder et al. 1997; Kucia et al. 2006d; He et al. 2007). In particular, the AGM region seems to be highly supportive for the origin, growth, maintenance and expansion of a variety of stem cells and progenitors such as endothelial stem cells (DeRuiter et al. 1997; Hatzopoulos et al. 1998; Ohneda et al. 1998; De Angelis et al. 1999; Condorelli et al. 2001), neural crest stem cells (Britsch et al. 1998; Moore and Larue 2004), mesoangioblasts (Minasi et al. 2002; Sampoalesi et al. 2003), haematopoietic progenitors (Jaffredo et al. 1998; Matsuoka et al. 2001; Oostendorp et al. 2002; Minasi et al. 2002; Tavian et al. 2005; Nobuhisa et al. 2007; Cumano and Godin 2007), primitive germ cells (Medvinsky et al. 1993; Hatano et al. 1996; He et al. 2007), prospective bone marrow stem cells (Minasi et al. 2002) and common steroidogenic progenitors for the adrenal gland and gonads (Luo et al. 1994; Sadovsky et al. 1995; Hatano et al. 1996; Morohashi 1997). Notably, the stroma of the urogenital ridge provides a highly supportive potential for HSCs (Oostendorp et al. 2002) and probably for other stem/progenitor cell types.

Chapter 9
Concluding Remarks

This monograph is devoted to the Leydig cells of rodent and human testes. In addition to reviewing the endocrine properties of the Leydig cells, we have paid particular attention to their striking, more recently established, neuroendocrine features. These features are stressed by the expression of a large number of neuroactive substances. Indicating importance for testis physiological function, some of these molecules are involved in the communication between neighbouring Leydig cells, Leydig and Sertoli cells, or Leydig cells and the testicular vasculature.

The question of the origin of the Leydig cells represents a second topic of this monograph. The identification of the neuroendocrine properties of the Leydig cells was the basis for and prompted us to search for their origin towards neuroectodermal or neural crest stem cell lineages. Using an experimental model to study the regenerative capacity of the Leydig cells in adult rats after their depletion by ethane dimethanesulphonate and by immunohistochemical analyses of the neural stem cell marker nestin, we were able to reveal that pericytes and smooth muscle cells of the testicular microvasculature serve as the stem/progenitor cells of all types of Leydig cells in the testis.

Pericytes (and vascular smooth muscle cells) do not express steroidogenic factors and enzymes which are characteristic for Leydig cells. Thus, the functional relationship between these cell types remained hidden for a long time. The discovered mode of transition of these vascular wall cells towards Leydig cells, in particular the process of transdifferentiation, was crucial to establishing the pericytes/smooth muscle cells as the precursors of the Leydig cells. In analogy to the nervous system, where the first progeny of neural stem cells is referred to as young neurons or neuroblasts, we propose designating the first members of the Leydig cell lineage as young Leydig cells because they are still able to divide before becoming amitotic adult Leydig cells. Remarkably, under certain exceptional conditions, even adult Leydig cells can be activated and do recover to a limited degree their capability to proliferate.

The Leydig cells show a remarkable association with the testicular microvasculature, which is evident during the whole life of an organism. Adult Leydig cells arise as descendants of blood vessel wall stem cells. An analogous functional interrelation seems to exist during embryonic testis development. Leydig cell development during this early period is closely associated with the formation of the testis-specific coelomic blood vessel. This vessel is assembled by mesonephros-derived endothelial stem cells and subsequently becomes stabilized by pericytes. The pericytes are either produced by the endothelial stem cells or acquired from pericyte progenitors located close by, presumably representing reticular stroma components of the aorta-gonad-mesonephros region known to contain a large number of different stem cell types.

In support of their role as stem cells for Leydig cells, pericytes (and vascular smooth muscle cells) are the only periendothelial cell types that are located within a true vascular stem cell niche, providing a basement membrane to these cells. Other perivascular cell types, including mesenchymal stem cells, are apart from the basement membrane and represent a heterogeneous cell population, also containing descendants of the pericytes, inclusive young or progenitor Leydig cells at different phases of their further differentiation. When such mesenchymal stem cells or progenitor cells are removed from their perivascular position and exposed to different environments, they can change their properties and produce a variety of progeny, including Leydig cell precursors.

Stem cells arising during early embryogenesis represent descendants of embryonal stem cells that generate a multifaceted progeny with qualities of both mesenchymal and neural lineages. Because the cardiovascular system is the first organ generated in the developing embryo and is indispensable for proper development and function of all other organ systems, pericyte progenitors and pericytes, recruited by endothelial cells and enclosed in the basal membrane of invading microvessels, may represent a lifelong reservoir of resting (silencing), early pluripotent stem cells for tissue repair and regeneration. In different organs, their fate (kind of progeny) depends on local, tissue-specific environmental factors.

At first glance, it seems intriguing that Leydig stem/progenitor cells and Leydig cells possess both mesodermal and neural properties. However, the results from investigations during the last 20 years have provided convincing evidence for this phenomenon. Taking into account that the germ layers of an embryo all arise from an earlier layer in the blastocyst (termed "epiblast") and that the embryonal mesoderm, the mesenchymal connective tissue, contains cells of the ectoderm, endoderm and mesoderm, an occurrence of early stem cells of the embryo that can produce a broad (mixed) progeny seems conceivable. This, however, questions the current theory on embryonic-layer-restricted stem cells. Recently, unique cells termed "very small embryonic-like stem cells" as well as mesenchymal-neural (mesectodermal) stem cells were discovered. Because these cells exhibit both mesodermal and neuroectodermal properties, it was proposed that they may be the common ancestors of both neural crest and mesenchymal stem cells. The features of the pericytes suggest their origin from early epiblast/ectodermal/neuroectodermal stem cells, and the identified lineage relationship with Leydig cells explains the multi- and pluripotent qualities of these cells.

Since fetal and adult Leydig cells are of the same origin, the phenotypic diversity of the Leydig cells during development and under different physiological and pathological conditions depends on the environmental factors in their vicinity. Generally, the Leydig cells behave as a remarkably stable cell population. Even in cases of the "Sertoli cell only syndrome", the Leydig cells survive and remain in the testis interstitium, where they support functions of the whole organism.

References

Abney TO, Myers RB (1991) 17ß-Estradiol inhibition of Leydig cell regeneration in the ethane dimethanesulfonate-treated mature rat. J Androl 12:295–304
Abney TO, Zhai J (1998) Gene expression of luteinizing hormone receptor and steroidogenic enzymes during Leydig cell development. J Mol Endocrinol 20:119–127
Adams IR, McLaren A (2002) Sexually dimorphic development of mouse primordial germ cells: switching from oogenesis to spermatogenesis. Development 129:1155–1164
Adams MI, Nock B, Truong R, Cicero TJ (1992) Nitric oxide control of steroidogenesis: endocrine effects of NG-nitro-L-arginine and comparisons to alcohol. Life Sci 50:PL35–PL40
Aguiari P, Leo S, Zavin B, Vindigni V, Rimessi A, Bianchi K, Franzin C, Corvito R, Rossato M, Vettor R, Abatangelo G, Pozzan T, Pinton P, Rizzuto R (2008) High glucose induces adipogenic differentiation of muscle-derived stem cells. Proc Natl Acad Sci USA 105:1226–1231
Alexanian AR, Sieber-Blum M (2003) Differentiating adult hippocampal stem cells into neural crest derivatives. Neuroscience 118:1–5
Alliot F, Rutin J, Leenen PJM, Pessac B (1999) Pericytes and periendothelial cells of brain parenchyma vessels co-express aminopeptidase N, aminopeptidase A, and nestin. J Neurosci Res 58:367–378
Almazan G, Vela JM, Molina-Holgado E, Guaza C (2001) Re-evaluation of nestin as a marker of oligodendrocyte lineage cells. Microsc Res Tech 52:753–765
Allt G, Lawrenson JG (2001) Pericytes: cell biology and pathology. Cells Tissues Organs 169:1–11
Alvarez-Buylla A, Garcia-Verdugo JM (2002) Neurogenesis in adult subventricular zone. J Neurosci 22:629–634
Alvarez-Buylla A, Lim DA (2004) For the long run: maintaining germinal niches in the adult brain. Neuron 41:683–686
Alvarez-Buylla A, Garcia-Verdugo JM, Tramontin AD (2001) A unified hypothesis on the lineage of neural stem cells. Nat Rev Neurosci 2:287–293
Ambrosino A, Russo D, Lamanna C, Assisi L, Rizzo M, Vittoria A, Cecio A (2003) Isoforms of nitric oxide syntahse in the pig testis. Acta Vet Brno 72:493–498
Amemiya T, Sasamura H, Mifune M, Kitamura Y, Hirahashi J, Hayashi M, Saruta T (1999) Vascular endothelial growth factor activates MAP kinase and enhances collagen synthesis in human mesangial cells. Kidney Int 56:2055–2063
Amoh Y, Li L, Yang M, Moossa AR, Katsuoka K, Penman S, Hoffman RM (2004) Nascent blood vessels in the skin arise from nestin-expressing hair-follicle cells. Proc Natl Acad Sci USA 101:12291–12295
Amoh Y, Li L, Katsuoka K, Penman S, Hoffman RM (2005a) Multipotent nestin-positive, keratin-negative hair-follicle bulge stem cells can form neurons. Proc Natl Acad Sci USA 102:5530–5534
Amoh Y, Li L, Campillo R, Kawahara K, Katsuoka K, Penman S, Hoffman RM (2005b) Implanted hair follicle stem cells form Schwann cells that support repair of severed peripheral nerves. Proc Natl Acad Sci USA 102:17734–17738

Amoureux MC, Cunningham BA, Edelman FM, Crassin KL (2000) N-CAM binding inhibits the proliferation of hippocampal progenitor cells and promotes their differentiation to a neuronal phenotype. J Neurosci 20:3631–3640

Anderson DJ (2001) Stem cells and pattern formation in the nervous system:the possible versus the actual. Neuron 30:19–35

Andreeva ER, Pugach IM, Gordon D, Orekhov AN (1998) Continuous subendothelial network formed by pericyte-like cells in human vascular bed. Tissue Cell 30:127–135

Angelova P, Davidoff MS (1989) Immunocytochemical demonstration of substance P in hamster Leydig cells during ontogenesis. Z Mikrosk Anat Forsch 103:560–566

Angelova P, Davidoff MS, Kanchev L (1991a) Substance P-induced inhibiting of Leydig cell steroidogenesis in primary culture. Andrologia 23:325–327

Angelova P, Davidoff MS, Kanchev L, Baleva-Ivanova K (1991b). Substance P: immunocytochemical localization and biological role in hamster gonads during ontogenesis. Funct Dev Morphol 1:3–8

Angelova P, Davidoff MS, Baleva K, Staykova M (1991c) Substance P and neuron-specific enolase-like immunoreactivity of rodent Leydig cells in tissue section and cell culture. Acta Histochem 91:131–139

Anjos-Afonso F, Bonnet D (2007) Nonhematopoietic/endothelial SSEA-1+ cells define the most primitive progenitors in the adult murine bone marrow mesenchymal compartment. Blood 109:1298–1306

Anversa P, Leri A, Kajstura J (2006b) Cardiac regeneration. J Am Coll Cardiol 47:1769–1776

Anversa P, Kajstura J, Leri A, Bolli R (2006a) Life and death of cardiac stem cells: a paradigm shift in cardiac biology. Circulation 113:1451–1463

Anversa P, Leri A, Rota M, Hosoda T, Bearzi C, Urbanek K, Kajstura J, Bolli R (2007) Concise review: stem cells, myocardial regeneration, and methodological artefacts. Stem Cells 25:589–601

Apte MV, Haber PS, Applegate TL, Norton ID, McCaghan GW, Korsten MA, Pirola RC, Wilson JS (2007) Periacinar stellate shaped cells in rat pancreas: identification, isolation, and culture. Gut 43:128–133

Ariyaratne HB, Mendis-Handagama SMLC (2000) Changes in the testis interstitium of Sprague Dawley rats from birth to sexual maturity. Biol Reprod 62:680–690

Ariyaratne HB, Mendis-Handagama SMLC, Hales DB, Mason JI (2000a) Studies on the onset of Leydig precursor cell differentiation in the prepubertal rat testis. Biol Reprod 63:165–171

Ariyaratne HB, Mason JI, Mendis-Handagama SMLC (2000b) Effects of thyroid and luteinizing hormones on the onset of precursor cell differentiation into Leydig progenitor cells in the prepubertal rat testis. Biol Reprod 63:898–904

Ariyaratne HB, Mendis-Handagama SMLC, Mason JI (2000c) Effects of tri-iodothyronine on testicular interstitial cells and androgen secretory capacity of the prepubertal rat. Biol Reprod 63:493–502

Ariyaratne S, Kim I, Mills N, Mason I, Mendis-Handagama C (2003) Effects of ethane dimethane sulfonate on the functional structure of the adult rat testis. Arch Androl 49:313–326

Armulik A, Abramsson A, Betsholtz C (2005) Endothelial/pericyte interactions Circ Res 97:512–523

Asakura A, Rudnicki MA, Komaki M (2001) Muscle satellite stem cells that exhibit myogenic, osteogenic, and adipogenic differentiation. Differentiation 68:245–253

Atanassova N, McKinnell C, Walker M, Turner KJ, Fisher JS, Morley M, Millar MR, Groome NP, Sharpe RM (1999) Permanent effects of neonatal estrogen exposure in rats on reproductive hormone levels, Sertoli cell number, and the efficiency of spermatogenesis in adulthood. Endocrinology 140:5364–5373

Atanassova N, McKinnell C, Turner KJ, Walker M, Fisher JS, Morley M, Millar MR, Groome NP, Sharpe RM (2000) Comparative effects of neonatal exposure of male rats to potent and weak (environmental) estrogens on spermatogenesis at puberty and the relationship to adult testis size and fertility: evidence for stimulatory effects of low estrogen levels. Endocrinology 141:3898–3907

Atanassova N, Koeva Y, Bakalska M, Pavlova E, Nikolov B, Davidoff M (2006) Loss and recovery of androgen receptor protein expression in the adult rat testis following androgen withdrawal by ethane dimethanesulfonate. Folia Histochem Cytochem 44:81–86

Ayer-LeLievre C, Olson L, Ebendal T, Hallböök F, Persson H (1988) Nerve growth factor mRNA and protein in the testis and epididymis of mouse and rat. Proc Natl Acad Sci USA 85:2628–2632

Bachem MG, Schneider E, Gross H, Weidenbach H, Schmid RM, Menke A, Siech M, Beger H, Grunert A, Adler G (1998) Identification, culture, and characterization of pancreatic stellate cells in rats and human. Gastroenterology 115:421–432

Bailey AS, Willenbring H, Jiang S, Anderson DA, Schroeder DA, Wong MH, Grompe M, Fleming WH (2006) Myeloid lineage progenitors give rise to vascular endothelium. Proc Natl Acad Sci USA 103:13156–13161

Bailey P, Holowacz T, Lassar AB (2001) The origin of skeletal muscle stem cells in the embryo and the adult. Curr Opin Cell Biol 13:679–689

Baloh R, Tansey MG, Lampe PA, Fahrner TJ, Enomoto H, Simburger KS, Leitner ML, Araki T, Johnson EM Jr, Milbrandt J (1998) Artemin, a novel member of the GDNF ligand family, supports peripheral and central nerons and signals through GFRa3-RET receptor complex. Neuron 21:1291–1302

Bakalska M, Atanassova N, Angelova P, Koeva Y, Nikolov B, Davidoff M (2001) Degeneration and restoration of spermatogenesis in relation to the changes in Leydig cell population following ethane dimethanesulfonate treatment in adult rats. Endocr Regul 35:209–215

Bakalska M, Atanassova N, Koeva Y, Nikolov B, Davidoff M (2004) Induction of male germ cell apoptosis by testosterone withdrawal after ethane dimethanesulfonate treatment in adult rats. Endocr Regul 38:103–110

Bakalska M, Atanassova N, Koeva Y, McKinnell C, Nikolov B, Davidoff M (2006) Quantification of germ cell apoptosis and survival in relation to renewal of Leydig cell population after EDS treatment of adult rats. Acta Morphol Anthropol 11:24–29

Baker PJ, O'Shaughnessy PJ (2001a) Role of gonadotrophins in regulating numbers of Leydig and Sertoli cells during fetal and postnatal development in mice. Reproduction 122:227–234

Balabanov R, Washington R, Wagnerova J, Dore-Duffy P (1996) CNS microvascular pericytes express macrophage-like function, cell surface integrin αM, and macrophage marker ED-2. Microvascular Res 52:127–142

Bardin CW (1996) Androgens: early attempts to evaluate Leydig cell function in man. In: Payne AH, Hardy MP, Russel LD (eds) The Leydig cell. Cache River, Vienna, pp 29–42

Bardin CW, Chen C-L C, Morris PL, Gerendai I, Boitani C, Liotta AS, Margioris A, Krieger DT (1987) Proopiomelanocortin-derived peptides in testis, ovary, and tissues of reproduction. Recent Prog Horm Res 43:1–28

Bartlett JM, Kerr JB, Sharpe RM (1986) The effect of selective destruction and regeneration of rat Leydig cells on the intratesticular distribution of testosterone and morphology of the seminiferous epithelium. J Androl 7:240–253

Bartlett JM, Weinbauer CF, Nieschlag E (1989a) Differential effect of FSH and testosterone on the maintenance of spermatogenesis in the adult hypophysectomized rat. J Endocrinol 121:49–58

Basciani S, Mariani S, Arizzi M, Ulisse S, Rucci N, Jannini EA, Rocca CD, Manicone A, Carani C, Spera G, Gnessi L (2002) Expression of platelet-drived growth factor-A (PDGF-A), PDGF-B, and PDGF receptor-α and -ß during human testicular development and disease. Clin Endocrinol Metab 87:2310–2319

Battula VL, Bareiss PM, Treml S, Conrad S, Albert I, Hojak S, Abele H, Schewe B, Just L, Skutella T, Bühring HJ (2007) Human placenta and bone marrow derived MSC cultured in serum-free, b-FGF-containing medium express cell surface frizzled-9 and SSEA-4 and give rise to multilineage differentiation. Differentiation 75:279–291

Bearzi C, Rota M, Hosoda T, Tillmanns J, Nascimbene A, De Angelis A, Yasizawa-Amano S, Trifonova I, Siggins RW, LeCapitane N, Cascapera S, Beltrami AP, D'Alessandro DA, Zias E, Quaini F, Urbanek K, Michler RE, Bolli R, Kajstura J, Leri A, Anversa P (2007) Human cardiac stem cells. Proc Natl Acad Sci USA 104:14068–14073

Beauchamp JR, Heslop L, Yu DSW, Tajbakhsh S, Kelly RG, Wernig A, Buckingham ME, Partridge TA, Zammit PS (2000) Expression of CD34 and Myf5 defines the majority of quiescent adult skeletal muscle satellite cells. J Cell Biol 151:1221–1233

Beckman JD, Grazul-Bilska AT, Johnson ML, Reynolds LP, Redmer DA (2006) Isolation and characterization of ovine luteal pericytes and effects of nitric oxide on pericyte expression of angiogenic factors. Endocrine 29:467–476

Behringer RR, Finegold MJ, Cate RL (1994) Müllerian inhibiting substanece function during mammalian sexual development. Cell 79:415–425

Beissner H (1898) Die Zwischensubstanz des Hodens und ihre Bedeutung. Arch Mikrosk Anat Entwicklungsmech 51:794–820

Belachew S, Chittajallu R, Aguierre AA, Yuan X, Kirby M, Anderson S, Gallo V (2003) Postnatal NG2 proteoglycan-expressing progenitor cells are intrinsically multipotent and generate functional neurons. J Cell Biol 161:169–186

Bendsen E, Byskov AG, Laursen SB, Larsen H-PE, Andersen CY, Westergaaed LG (2003) Number of germ cells and somatic cells in human fetal testes during the first weeks after sex differentiation. Hum Reprod 18:13–18

Benton L, Shan L-X, Hardy MP (1995) Differentiation of adult Leygig cells. J Steroid Biochem Mol Biol 53:61–68

Benvenuti S, Luciani P, Cellai I, Deledda C, Baglioni S, Saccardi R, Urbani S, Francini F, Squecco R, Guiliani C, Vanelli GB, Serio M, Pinchera A, Peri A (2008) Thyroid hormones promote cell differentiation and up-regulate the expression of the seladin-1 gene in in vitro models of human neuronal precursors. J Endocrinol 197:437–446

Ben-Yair R, Kalcheim C (2008) Notch and bone morphogenetic protein differentially act on dermomyotome cells to generate endothelium, smooth, and striated muscle. J Cell Biol 180:607–618

Bergers G, Song S (2005) The role of pericytes in blood-vessel formation and maintenance. Neuro-oncology 7:452–464

Bergh A (1982) Local differences in Leydig cell morphology in the adult rat testis: evidence for a local control of Leydig cells by the adjacent seminiferous tubules. Int J Androl 5:325–330

Bergh A (1983) Paracrine regulation of Leydig cell morphology in the adult testis: evidence for a local control of Leydig cells by the adjacent seminiferous tubules. Int J Androl 6:57–65

Bergh A, Damber JE (1992) Immunohistochemical demonstration of androgen receptors on testicular blood vessels. Int J Androl 15:425–434

Bergwerff M, Verberene ME, DeRuiter MC, Poelmann RE, Gittenberger-de Groot AC (1998) Neural crest cell contribution to the developing circulatory system. Implications for vascular morphology? Circ Res 82:221–231

Berthold AA (1849a) Transplatation der Hoden. Arch Anat Physiol Wiss Med 16:42–46

Berthold AA (1849b) Über die Transplantation der Hoden. Nachr K Ges Wiss 1:1–6

Bianco P, Cossu G (1999) Uno, nessuno e centromila: searching for the identity of mesodermal progenitors. Exp Cell Res 251:257–263

Bianco P, Robey PG (2000) Marrow stromal stem cells. J Clin Invest 105:1663–1668

Bianco P, Riminucci M, Gronthos S, Robey PG (2001) Bone marrow stromal cells: nature, biology, and potential applications. Stem Cells 19:180–192

Billon N, Innarelli P, Monteiro MC, Glavieux-Pardanaud C, Richardson WD, Kessaris N, Dani C, Dupin E (2007) The generation of adipocytes by the neural crest. Development 134:2283–2292

Bilinska B (1989) Visualization of the cytoskeleton in Leydig cells in vitro. Histochemistry 93:105–110

Bishop CE, Whitworth DJ, Qin Y, Agoulnik AI, Agoulnik IU, Harison WR, Behringer RR, Oberbeek RA (2000) A transgenic insertion upstream of Sox9 is associated with dominant XX sex reversal in the mouse. Nat Genet 26:490–494

Biswas A, Hutchins R (2007) Embryonic stem cells. Stem Cells Dev 16:213–221

Bitgood MJ, Shen L, McMahon AP (1996) Sertoli cell signaling by Desert hedgehog regulates the male germline. Curr Biol 6:298–304

Bixby S, Kruger GM, Mosher JT, Joseph NM, Morrison SJ (2002) Cell-intrinsic differences between stem cells from different regions of the peripheral nervous system regulate the generation of neural diversity. Neuron 35:643–656

Bjornson CRR, Rietze RL, Reynolds BA, Magli MC, Vescovi AL (1999) Turning brain into blood: a hematopoietic fate adopted by adult neural stem cells in vivo. Science 283:534–537

Blanpain C, Fuchs E (2006) Epidermal stem cells of the skin. Annu Rev Cell Dev Biol 22:339–373

Blanpain C, Lowry WE, Geoghegan A, Polak L, Fuchs E (2004) Self-renewal, multipotency, and the existence of two populations within an epiphyseal stem cell niche. Cell 118:635–648

Boll F (1869) Beiträge zur mikroskopischen Anatomie der azinösen Drüsen (according to Beissner 1898)

Boll (1871) Untersuchungen über den Bau und die Entwicklung der Gewebe. Arch Mikrosk Anat 7:322

Bondjers C, Kalen M, Hellström M, Scheidl SJ, Abramsson A, Renner O, Lindahl P, Cho H, Kehrl J, Betsholtz C (2003) Transcription profiling of platelet-derived growth factor-B-deficient mouse embryos identifies RGS5 as a novel marker for pericytes and vascular smooth muscle cells. Am J Pathol 162:721–729

Bondjers C, He L, Takemoto M, Norlin J, Asker N, Hellström M, Lindahl P, Betsholtz C (2006) Microarray analysis of blood microvessels from PDGF-B and PDGF-Rß mutant mice identifies novel markers for brain pericytes. FASEB J 20:E1005–1013

Bondurand N, Natarajan D, Thapar N, Atkins C, Pachnis V (2003) Neuron and glia generating progenitors in the mammalian enteric nervous system isolated from foetal and postnatal gut cultures. Development 130:6387–6400

Botham CA, Jones GV, Kendall MD (2001) Immuno-characterization of neuroendocrine cells of the rat thymus gland in vitro and in vivo. Cell Tissue Res 303:381–389

Bouin P, Ancel P (1903) Recherches sur les cellules interstitielles du testicule des mammifères. Arch Zool Exp Gen 4 Ser 1:437–523

Bouin P, Ancel P (1904) La glande interstitielle a seule, dans le testicle, une action générale sur l'organisme. Démonstration expérimentale. C R Acad Sci 138:110–112

Bowles J, Knight D, Smith C, Wilhelm D, Richman J, Mamiya S, Yashiro H, Chawengsaksophak K, Wilson MJ, Rossant J, Hamada H, Koopman P (2006) Retinoic signalling determines germ cell fate in mice. Science 312:596–600

Brand-Saberi B, Christ B (2000) Evolution and development of distinct cell lineages derived from somites. Curr Top Dev Biol 48:1–42

Bremner WJ, Millar MR, Sharpe RM, Saunders PTK (1994) Immunohistochemical localization of androgen receptors in the rat testis: evidence for stage-dependent expression and regulation by androgens. Endocrinology 135:1227–1234

Brennan J, Capel B (2004) One tissue, two fates: molecular genetic events that underlie testis versus ovary development. Nat Rev Gen 5:509–521

Brennan J, Karl J, Capel B (2002) Divergent vascular mechanisms downstream of Sry establish the arterial system in the XY gonad. Dev Biol 244:418–428

Brennan J, Tilmannn C, Capel B (2003) Pdgfr-α mediates testis cord organization and fetal Leydig cell development in the XY gonad. Genes Dev 17:800–810
Britsch S, Li L, Kirchhoff S, Theuring F, Brinkmann V, Birchmeier C, Riethmacher D (1998) The ErbB2 and ErbB3 receptors and their ligand, neuregulin-1, are essential for development of the sympathetic nervous system. Genes Dev 12:1825–1836
Buehr M, Gu S, McLaren A (1993) Mesonephric contribution to testis differentiation in the fetal mouse, Development 117:273–281
Burnett AL (1995) Role of nitric oxide in the physiology of erection. Biol Reprod 52:485–489
Bühring HJ, Battula VL, Treml S, Schewe L, Kanz L, Vogel W (2007) Novel markers for the prospective isolation of human MSC. Ann N Y Acad Sci 1106:263–271
Byskov AG (1986) Differentiation of mammalian embryonic gonad. Phys Rev 66:71–117
Callard (1996) Endocrinology of Leydig cells in nonmammalian vertebrates. In: Payne AH, Hardy MP, Russel LD (eds) The Leydig cell. Cache River, Vienna, pp 307–332
Calloni GW, Glavieux-Pardanaud C, Le Douarin NM, Dupin E (2007) Sonic hedgehog promotes the development of multipotent neural crest progenitors endowed with both mesenchymal and neural potentials. Proc Natl Acad Sci USA 104:19879–19884
Campa VM, Gutiérez-Lanza R, Cerignoli F, Diaz-Trelles R, Nelson B, Tsuji T, Bracova M, Jiang W, Mercola M (2008) Notch activates cell cycle reentry and progression in quiescent cardiomyocytes. J Cell Biol 183:129–141
Cao L, Jiao X, Zuzga DS, Liu Y, Fong DM, Young D, During MJ (2004) VEGF links hippocampal activity with neurogenesis, learning and memory. Nat Gen 36:827–835
Capel B, Albrecht KH, Washburn LL, Eicher EM (1999) Migration of mesonephric cells into mammalian gonad depends on Sry. Mech Dev 84:127–131
Carlson SH, Wyss JM (2008) Neurohormonal regulation of the sympathetic nervous system: new insights into central mechanisms of action. Curr Hypertens Res 10:233–240
Carmeliet P (2000) One cell, two fates. Nature 408:43–45
Carmeliet P (2003) Blood vessels and nerves: common signals, pathways and diseases. Nat Gen 4:710–720
Carmeliet P, Tessier-Lavigne M (2005) Common mechanisms of nerve and blood vessel wiring. Nature 436:193–200
Carreau S (2007) Leydig cell aromatase. In: Payne AH, Hardy MP (eds) Contemporarry endocrinology: the Leydig cell in health and disease. Humana, Totowa, pp 189–195
Carreau S, de Vienne C, Galeraud-Denis I (2008) Aromatase and estrogens in man reproduction: a review and latest advances. Adv Med Sci 53:139–144.
Cassiman D, van Pelt J, De Vos R, VanLommel F, Desmet V, Yap SH, Roskams T (1999) Synaptophysin: a novel marker for human and rat hepatic stellate cells. Am J Pathol 155:1831–1839
Cassiman D, Denef C, Desmet VJ, Roskams T (2001) Human and rat hepatic stellate cells express neurotrophins and neurotrophin receptors. Hepathology 33:148–158
Cassiman D, Libbrecht L, Desmet V, Denef C, Roskams T (2002) Hepatic stellate cell/myofibroblast subpopulations in fibrotic human and rat livers. J Hepatol 36:200–209
Cassiman D, Sinelli N, Bockx I, Vander Borght S, Petersen B, De Vos B, van Pelt J, Nevens F, Libbrecht L, Roskams T (2007) Human hepatic progenitor cells express vasoactive intestinal peptide receptor type 2 and receive nerve endings. Liver Int 27:323–328
Chai Y, Jiang X, Ito Y, Bringas P Jr, Han J, Rowitch DH, Soriano P, McMahon AP, Sucov HM (2000) Fate of mammalian cranial neural crest during tooth and mandibular morphogenesis. Development 127:1671–1679
Chakravarthy B, Rashid A, Brown L, Tessier L, Kelly J, Ménard M (2008) Association of Gap-43 (neuromodulin) with microtubule-associated protein MAP-2 in neuronal cells. Biochem Biophys Res Commun 371:679–683

Chandrashekar V, Bartke A (2007) Growth factors in Leydig cell functions. In: Payne AH, Hardy MP (eds) Contemporarry endocrinology: the Leydig cell in health and disease. Humana, Totowa, pp 263–277

Chang E, Yang J, Nagavarupu U, Herron GS (2002) Aging of cutaneous microvasculature. J Invest Dermatol 118:752–758

Chemes HE (1996) Leydig cell development in humans. In: Payne AH, Hardy MP, Russel LD (eds) The Leydig cell. Cache River, Vienna, pp 175–201

Chemes H, Gigorraga S, Bergadá C, Schteingart H, Rev R, Pellizzari E (1992) Isolation of human Leydig cell mesenchymal precursors from patients with the androgen insensitivity syndrome: testosterone production and response to human chorionic gonadotropin stimulation in culture. Biol Reprod 46:793–801

Chen C-LC, Mather JP, Morris PL, Bardin CW (1984) Expression of proopiomelanocortin-like gene in testis and epididymis. Proc Natl Acad Sci USA 81:5672–5675

Chen H, Huhtaniemi I, Zirkin BR (1996a) Depletion and repopulation of Leydig cells in the testes of aging brown norvay rats. Endocrinology 137:3447–3452

Chen H, Luo L, Zirkin BR (1996b) Leydig cell structure and function during aging. In: Payne AH, Hardy MP, Russell LD (eds) The Leydig cell. Cache River, Vienna, pp 221–230

Chen H, Midzak A, Luo L-di, Zirkin BR (2007) Aging and the decline of androgen production. In: Payne AH, Hardy MP (eds) Contemporarry endocrinology: the Leydig cell in health and disease. Humana, Totowa, pp 117–131

Chen SC, Marino V, Gronthos S, Bartold PM (2006) Location of putative stem cells in human periodontal ligament. J Periodont Res 41:547–553

Chiquoine AD (1954) The identification, origin, and migration of the primordial germ cells in the mouse embryo. Anat Rec 118:135–146

Chiwakata C, Brackmann , Hunt N, Davidoff M, Schulze W, Ivell R (1991) Tachykinin (Substance P) gene expression in Leydig cells of the human and mouse testis. Endocrinology 128:2441–1448

Cho H, Kozasa T, Bondjers C, Betsholtz C, Kehrl JH (2003) Pericyte-specific expression of Rgs5: implications for PDGF and EDG receptor signalling during vascular maturation. FASEB J 17:440–442

Christ B, Huang R, Scaal M (2004) Formation and differentiation of the avian somite. Anat Embryol 208:333–350

Christensen AK (1965) Fine structure of testicular interstitial cells in guinea pigs. J Cell Biol 26:911–935

Christensen AK (1970) Fine structure of testicular interstitial cells in humans. In: Rosemberg E, Paulsen CA (eds) The human testis. Plenum, New York, pp 75–93

Christensen AK (1975) Leydig cells. In: Hamilton DW, Greep RO (eds) Male reproductive system. Am Physiol Soc V:57–94

Christensen AK (1996) A history of studies on testicular Leydig cells: the first century. In: Payne AH, Hardy MP, Russell LD (eds) The Leydig cell. Cache River, Vienna, pp 1–29

Christensen AK (2007) A history of Leydig cell research. In: Payne AH, Hardy MP (eds) Contemporarry endocrinology: the Leydig cell in health and disease. Humana, Totowa, pp 3–30

Christensen AK, Mason NR (1965) Comparative ability of seminiferous tubules and interstitial tissue of rat testis to synthesize androgens from progesterone-4-14C in vitro. Endocrinology 76:646–656

Ciampani I, Fabbri A, Isidori A, Dufau ML (1992) Growth hormone-releasing hormone is produced by rat Leydig cell in culture and acts as a positive regulator of Leydig cell function. Endocrinology 131:2785–2792

Clark AM, Garland KK, Russell LD (2000) Desert hedgehog (Dhh) gene is required in the mouse testis for formation of adult-type Leydig cells and normal development of peritubular cells and seminiferous tubules. Biol Reprod 63:1825–1838

Clarke DL, Johansson CB, Wilbertz J, Veress B, Nilsson E, Karlström J, Lendahl U, Frisén J (2000) Generalized potential of adult neural stem cells. Science 288:1660–1663
Clegg EJ, Macmillan EW (1965) The phagocytic nature of Schiff-positive interstitial cells in the rat testis. J Endocrinol 31:299–300
Collesi C, Zentlin L, Sinagra G, Giacca M (2008) Notch1 signaling stimulates proliferation of immature cardiomyocytes. J Cell Biol 183:117–128
Collin O, Bergh A (1996) Leydig cells secrete factors which increase vascular permeability and endothelial cell proliferation. Int J Androl 19:221–228
Colvin JS, Green RP, Schmahl J, Capel B, Ornitz DM (2001) Male-to-female sex reversal in mice lacking fibroblast growth factor 9. Cell 104:875–889
Condorelli G, Borello U, De Angelis L, Latronico M, Sirabella D, Coletta M, Galli R, Balconi G, Follenzi A, Frati G, Cusella de Angelis MG, Gioglio L, Amuchastegui S, Adorini L, Naldini L, Vescovi A, Decana E, Cossu G (2001) Cardiomyocytes induce endothelial cells to transdifferentiate into cardiac muscle: implications for myocardium regeneration. Proc Natl Acad Sci USA 98:10733–10738
Cooke BA, Choi MCK, Dirami G, Lopez-Ruiz MP, West AP (1992) Control of steroidogenesis in Leydig cells. J Steroid Biochem Mol Biol 43:445–449
Cool J, Carmona FD, Szucsik JC, Capel B (2008) Peritubular myoid cells are not the migrating population required for testis cord formation in the XY gonad. Sex Dev 2:128–133
Cossu G, Bianco P (2003) Mesoangioblasts – vascular progenitors for extravascular mesodermal tissues. Curr Opin Genet Dev 13:537–542
Covas DT, Panepussi RA, Fontes AM, Silva WA Jr, Orellana MD, Freitas MCC, Neder L, Santos ARD, Peres LC, Jamur MC, Zago MA (2008) Multipotent mesenchymal stromal cells obtained from diverse human tissues share functional properties and gene-expression profile with CD146+ perivascular cells and fibroblasts. Exp Hematol 36:642–654
Coveney D, Cool J, Capel B (2008) Four-dimensional analysis of vascularization during primary development of an organ, the gonad. Proc Natl Acad Sci USA 105:7212–7217
Coyne TM, Marcus AJ, Woodbury D, Black IB (2006) Marrow stromal cells transplanted to the adult brain are rejected by an inflamatory response and transfer donor labels to host neurons and glia. Stem Cells 24:2483–2492
Crane JF, Trainor PA (2006) Neural crest stem and progenitor cells. Annu Rev Cell Dev Biol 22:267–286
Cui S, Schwartz L, Qiaggin SE (2003) Pod1 is required in stromal cells for glomerulogenesis. Dev Dyn 226:512–522
Cui S, Ross A, Stallings N, Parker KL, Capel B, Quaggin SE (2004) Disrupted gonadogenesis and male-to-female sex reversal in Pod1 knockout mice. Development 131:4095–4105
Cumano A, Godin I (2007) Ontogeny of the hematopoietic system. Annu Rev Immunol 25:745–785
Dabeva MD, Shafritz DA (1993) Activation, proliferation, and differentiation of progenitor cells into hepatocytes in the D-galactosamine model of liver regeneration. Am J Pathol 143:1606–1620
Dabeva MD, Hwang S-G, Vasa SRG, Hurston E, Novikoff PM, Hixon DC, Gupta S, Shafritz DA (1997) Differentiation of pancreatic epithelial progenitor cells into hepatocytes following transplantation into rat liver. Proc Natl Acad Sci USA 94:7356–7361
D'Alessandro JS, Lu K, Fung BP, Colman A, Clarke DL (2007) Rapid and efficient in vitro generation of pancreatic islet progenitor cells from nonendocrine epithel cells in the adult human pancreas. Stem Cells Dev 16:75–89
Danet GH, Luongo JL, Butler G, Lu MM, Tenner AJ, Simon MC, Bonnet DA (2002) C1qRp defines a new human stem cell population with hematopoietic and hepatic potential. Proc Natl Acad Sci USA 99:10441–10445

Dahlstrand J, Zimmerman LB, McKay RDG, Lendahl U (1992a) Characterization of the human nestin gene reveals a close evolutionary relationship to neurofilaments. J Cell Sci 103:589–597

Dahlstrand J, Collins VP, Lendahl U (1992b) Expression of the class VI intermediate filament nestin in human central nervous system tumors. Cancer Res 52:5334–5341

Dahlstrand J, Lardelli M, Lendahl U (1995) Nestin mRNA expression correlates with the CNS progenitor cell state in many, but not all, regions of developing CNS. Dev Brain Res 84:109–129

Darland DC, D'Amore PA (2001) TGF beta is required for the formation of capillary-like structures in three-dimensional cocultures of 10T1/2 and endothelial cells. Angiogenesis 4:11–20

Darland DC, Massingham LJ, Smith SR, Piek E, Saint-Geniez M, D'Amore PA (2003) Pericyte production of cell-associated VEGF is differentiation-dependent and is associated with endothelial survival. Dev Biol 264:275–288

Darlington PJ, Goldman JS, Ciu Q-I, Antel JP, Kennedy TE (2008) Widespread immunoreactivity for neuronal nuclei in cultured human and rodent astrocytes. J Neurochem 104:1201–1209

da Silva Meirelles L, Chagastelles PC, Nardi NB (2006) Mesenchymal stem cells reside in virtually all post-natal organs and tissues. J Cell Sci 119:2204–2213

da Silva Meirelles L, Caplan AI, Nardi NB (2008) In serch of the in vivo identity of mesenchymal stem cells. Stem Cells 26:2287–2299

David K (1935) Über das Testosteron, das kristallisierte männliche Hormon aus Stierentestes. Acta Brevia Neerl 5:85–108

David K, Dingemanse E, Freud J, Laqueur E (1935) Über krystallinisches männliches Hormon aus Hoden (Testosteron), wirksamer als aus Harn oder aus Cholesterin bereitetes Androsteron. Z Phys Chem 233:281–282

Davidoff M (1986) Immunocytochemistry – possibilities for demonstration of different tissue antigens and establishment of the functional role of cells. Acta Histochem 33(Suppl):175–193

Davidoff M, Schulze W (1990) Combination of the peroxidase anti-peroxidase (PAP)- and avidin-biotin-peroxidase complex (ABC)-tchniques: an amplification alternative in immunocytochemical staining. Histochemistry 93:531–536

Davidoff MS, Middendorff R (2000) The nitric oxide sytsem in the urogenital tract. In: Steinbusch HWM, de Vente J, Vincent S (eds) Functional neuroanatomy of the nitric oxide system. Handbook of chemical neuroanatomy, vol 17. Elsevier, Amsterdam, pp 267–314

Davidoff MS, Breucker H, Holstein AF, Seidel K (1990) Cellular architecture of the lamina propria of human seminiferous tubules. Cell Tissue Res 262:253–261

Davidoff MS, Schulze W, Middendorff R, Holstein AF (1993) The Leydig cell of the human testis – a new member of the diffuse neuroendocrine system. Cell Tissue Res 271:429–439

Davidoff MS, Middendorff R, Mayer B, Holstein AF (1995) Nitric oxide synthase (NOS-1) in Leydig cells of the human testis. Arch Histol Cytol 58:17–30

Davidoff MS, Middendorff R, Holstein AF (1996) Dual nature of Leydig cells of the human testis. Biomed Rev 6:11–41

Davidoff MS, Middendorff R, Mayer B, de Vente J, Koesling D, Holstein AF (1997a) Nitric oxide/cGMP-pathway components in Leydig cells of the human testis. Cell Tissue Res 287:161–170

Davidoff MS, Middendorff R, Müller D, Köfüncü E, Holstein AF (1997b) Immunoreactivity for glial cell markers in the human testis. Adv Exp Med Biol 424:151–152

Davidoff MS, Middendorff R, Pusch W, Müller D, Wichers S, Holstein AF (1999) Sertoli and Leydig cells of the human testis express neurofilament triplet proteins. Histochem Cell Biol 111:173–187

Davidoff MS, Middendorff R, Koeva Y, Pusch W, Jezek D, Müller D (2001) Glial cell line-derived neurotrophic factor (GDNF) and its receptors GFRα-1 and GFRα-2 in the human testis. Ital J Anat Embryol 106(Suppl 2):173–180

Davidoff MS, Middendorff R, Köfüncü E, Müller D, Ježek D, Holstein AF (2002) Leydig cells of the human testis possess astrocyte and olygodendrocyte marker molecules. Acta Histochem 104:39–49

Davidoff MS, Middendorff R, Enikolopov G, Riethmacher D, Holstein AF, Müller D (2004) Progenitor cells of the testosterone-producing Leydig cells revealed. J Cell Biol 167:935–944

Davidoff MS, Ungefroren U, Middendrorff R, Koeva Y, Bakalska M, Atanassova N, Holstein AF, Ježek D, Pusch W, Müller D (2005) Catecholamine-synthesizing enzymes in the adult and prenatal human testis. Histochem Cell Biol 124:313–323

Dawson VL (1995) Nitric oxide: role in neurotoxicity. Clin Exp Pharmacol Physiol 22:305–308

Day K, Shefer G, Richardson JB, Enikolopov G, Yablonka-Reuveni Z (2007) Nestin-GFP reporter expression defines the quiescent state of skeletal muscle satellite cells. Dev Biol 304:246–259

De Angelis L, Berghella L, Coletta M, Lattanzi L, Zanchi M, Cusella-De Angelis MG, Ponzetto C, Cossu G (1999) Skeletal myogenic progenitors originating from embryonic dorsal aorta coexpress endothelial and myogenic markers and contribute to postnatal muscle growth and regeneration. J Cell Biol 147:869–877

Debeljuk L, Rao JN, Bartke A (2003) Tachykinins and their possible modulatory role on testicular function: a review. Int J Androl 26:202–210

De Gendt K, Atanassova N, Tan KAL, de França LR, Perreira GG, McKinnell, Sharpe RM, Saunders PTK, Mason JI, Hartung S, Ivell R, Denolet E, Verhoeven G (2005) Development and function of adult generation of Leydig cells in mice with Sertoli cell-selective or total ablation of the androgen receptor. Endocrinology 146:4117–4126

De Groat WC, Kawatani M, Hisamitsu T, Lowe I, Morgan R, Rappolo J, Booth AM, Nadelhaft I, Kuo D, Thork K (1983) The role of neuropeptides in the sacral autonomic reflex pathways of the cat. J Auton Nerv Syst 7:339–350

de Kretser DM (1982) Sertoli cell-Leydig cell interaction in the regulation of testicular function. Int J Androl 5(Suppl):11–17

de Kretser DM (1987) Local regulation of testicular function. Int Rev Cytol 109:89–112

de Kretser DM, Kerr JB (1994) The cytology of the testis. In: Knobil E, Neill JD (eds) The physiology of reproduction, vol 1, 2nd edn. Raven, New York, pp 1177–1290

Delbès G, Levacher C, Ducuenne C, Racine C, Pakarinen P, Habert R (2005) Endogenous estrogens inhibit mouse fetal Leydig cell development via estrogen receptor α. Endocrinology 146:2454–2461

Dellavalle A, Sampaolesi M, Tonlorenzi R, Tagliafico E, Sacchetti B, Pearni L, Innocenzi A, Galvez BG, Messina G, Morosseti R, Sheng Li, Belicchi M, Peretti G, Chamberlain JS, Wright WE, Torrente Y, Ferrari S, Bianco P, Gossu G (2007) Pericytes of human skeletal muscle are myogenic precursors distinct from satellite cells. Nat Cell Biol 9:255–267

Del Punta K, Charreau EH, Pignataro OP (1996) Nitric oxide inhibits Leydig cell steroidogenesis. Endocrinology 137:5337–5343

Deng J, Steindler DA, Laywell ED, Petersen BE (2003) Neural trans-differentiation potential of hepatic oval cells in the neonatal mouse brain. Exp Neurol 182:373–382

DeRuiter MC, Poelmann RE, VanMunsteren JC, Mironov V, Markwald RR, Gittenberg-de Groot AC (1997) Embryonic endothelial cells transdifferentiate into mesenchymal cells expressing smooth muscle actins in vivo and in vitro. Circ Res 80:444–451

Deschepper CF, Mellon SH, Cumin F, Baxter JD, Ganong WF (1986) Analysis by immunocylochemistry and in situ hybridization of renin and its mRNA in kidney, testis, adrenal, and pituitary of the rat. Proc Natl Acad Sci USA. 83:7552–7556

DiNapoli L, Capel B (2008) SRY and the standoff in sex determination. Mol Endocrinol 22:1–9

DiNapoli L, Batchvarov J, Capel B (2006) FGF9 promotes survival of germ cells in the fetal testis. Development 133:1519–1527
Doepner RFG, Geigerseder C, Frungieri MB, Gonzalez-Calvar SI, Calandra RS, Raemsch R, Föhr K, Kunz L, Mayerhofer A (2005) Insights into GABA receptor signalling in TM3 Leydig cells. Neuroendocrinology 81:381–390
Doetsch F (2003a) The glial identity of neural stem cells. Nature Neurosci 6:1127–1134
Doetsch F (2003b) A niche for adult neural stem cells. Curr Opin Genet Dev 13:543–550
Doetsch F, Caille I, Lim DA, Garcia-Verdugo JM, Alvarez-Buylla A (1999a) Subventricular zone astrocytes are neural stem cells in the adult mammalian brain. Cell 97:703–716
Doetsch F, Garcia-Verdugo JM, Alvarez-Buylla A (1999b) Regeneration of a germinal layer in the adult mammalian brain. Proc Natl Acad Sci USA 96:11619–11624
Doherty MJ, Ashton BA, Walsh S, Beresford JN, Grant ME, Canfield AE (1998) Vascular pericytes express osteogenic potential in vitro and in vivo. J Bone Miner Res 13:828–838
Dominici M, Pritchard C, Garlits JE, Hofmann TJ, Persons DA, Horwitz EM (2004) Hematopoietic cells and osteoblasts are derived from a common marrow progenitor after bone marrow transplantation. Proc Natl Acad Sci USA 101:11761–11766
Dong L, Jelinsky SA, Finger JN, Johnston DS, Korf GS, Sottas CM, Hardy MP, Ge R-S (2007) Gene expression during development of fetal and adult Leydig cells. Ann N Y Acad Sci 1120:16–35
Dore-Duffy P, Owen C, Balabanov R, Murphy S, Beaumont T, Rafols JA (2000) Pericyte migration from the vascular wall in response to traumatic brain injury. Microvasc Res 60:55–69
Dore-Duffy P, Katychev A, Wang X, Van Buren E (2006) CNS microvascular pericytes exhibit multipotential stem cell activity. J Cereb Blood Flow Metab 26:613–624
Doyle B, Matharom P, Caplice NM (2006) Endothelial progenitor cells. Endothelium 13:403–410
Drusenheimer N, Wulf G, Nolte J, Lee JH, Dev A, Dressel R, Gromoll J, Schmidtke J, Engel W, Nayernia K (2007) Putative human male germ cells from bone marrow stem cells. Soc Reprod Fertil Suppl 63:69–76
Du J, Hull EM (1999) Effects of testosterone on neuronal nitric oxide synthase and tyrosine hydroxylase. Brain Res 836:90–98
Dufau ML, Tsai-Morris C-H (2007) The luteinizing hormone receptor. In: Payne AH, Hardy MP (eds) Contemporarry endocrinology: the Leydig cell in health and disease. Humana, Totowa, 227–252
Dupin E, Calloni G, Real C, Gonçalves-Trentin A, Le Douarin NM (2007) Neural crest progenitor and stem cells. C R Biol 330:521–529
Dupont É, Labrie F, Luu-The V, Pelletier G (1993) Ontogeny of 3ß-hydroxysteroid dehydrogenase/Δ-5-Δ4 isomerase (3ß-HSD) in rat testis as studied by immunocytochemistry. Anat Embryol 187:583–589
Durcova-Hills G, Adams IR, Barton SC, Surani MA, McLaren A (2006) The role of exogenous fibroblast growth factor-2 on the reprogramming of primordial germ cells into pluripotent stem cells. Stem Cells 24:1441–1449
Ehler E, Karlhuber C, Bauer H-C, Draeger A (1995) Heterogeneity of smooth muscle-associated proteins in mammalian brain microvasculature. Cell Tissue Res 279:393–403
El-Gehani F, Tena-Sempere M, Ruskoaho H, Huhtaniemi I (2001) Natriuretic peptides stimulate steroidogenesis in the fetal rat testis. Biol Reprod 65:595–600
Ergün S, Stingl J, Holstein AF (1994a) Segmental angioarchitecture of the testicular lobule in man. Andrologia 26:143–150
Ergün S, Stingl J, Holstein AF (1994b) Microvasculature of the human testis in correlation to Leydig cells and seminiferous tubules. Andrologia 26:255–262
Ergün S, Davidoff M, Holstein AF (1996) Capillaries in the lamina propria of human seminiferous tubules are partly fenestrated. Cell Tissue Res 286:93–102

Ergün S, Kiliç N, Fiedler W, Mukhopadhyay AK (1997) Vascular endothelial growth factor and its receptors in normal human testicular tissue. Mol Cell Endocrinol 131:9–20

Ergün S, Harneit S, Paust HJ, Mukhopadhyay AK, Holstein AF (1999) Endothelin and endothelin receptors A and B in the human testis. Anat Embryol 199:207–214

Esner M, Meilhac SM, Relaix F, Nicolas J-F, Cossu G, Buckingam ME (2006) Smooth muscle of the dorsal aorta shares a common clonal origin with skeletal muscle of the myotome. Development 133:737–749

Ewing JF, Maincs MD (1995) Distribution of constitutive (HO-2) and heat-inducible (HO-1) heme oxygenase isozymes in rat testis: HO-2 displays stage-specific expression in germ cells. Endocrinology 136:2294–2302

Fabbri A, Knox G, Buczko E, Dufau ML (1988) Beta-endorphin production by the fetal Leydig cells: regulation and implications for paracrine control of Sertoli cell function. Endocrinology 122:749–755

Fabel K, Fabel K, Tam B, Kaufer D, Baiker A, Simmons N, Kuo CJ, Palmer TD (2003) VEGF is necessary for exercise-induced adult hippocampal neurogenesis. Eur J Neurosci 18:2803–2812

Farrington-Rock C, Crofts NJ, Doherty MJ, Ashton BA, Griffin-Jones C, Canfield AE (2004) Chondrogenic and adipogenic potential of microvascular pericytes. Circulation 110:2226–2232

Fecteau KA, Mrkonjich L, Mason JI, Mendis-Handagama SMLC (2006) Detection of platelet-derived growth factor-alpha (PDGF-A) protein in cells of Leydig lineage in the postnatal rat testis. Histol Histopathol 21:1295–1302

Feng P, Carnell NE, Kim UJ, Jacobs S, Wilber JF (1992) The human testis: a novel locus for thyrotropin-rceasing hormone (TRH) and TRH mRNA. Trans Assoc Am Physicians 105:222–228

Fernandes KJL, Toma JG, Miller FD (2008) Multipotent skin-derived precursors: adult neural crest-related precursors with therapeutic potential. Philos Trans R Soc B 363:185–198

Ferrara N, Gerber H-P, LeCouter J (2003) The biology of VEGF and its receptors. Nat Med 9:669–676

Ferrara N, LeCouter J, Lin R, Peale F (2004) EG-VEGF and Bv8: a novel family of tissue-restricted angiogenic factors. Biochim Biophys Acta 1654:69–78

Ferrari G, Cusella-De Angelis G, Coletta M, Paolucci E, Stornaiuolo A, Cossu G, Mavilio M (1998) Muscle regeneration by bone marrow-derived myogenic progenitors. Science 279:1528–1530

Foster K, Sheridan J, Veiga-Fernandes H, Roderick K, Pachnis V, Adams R, Blackburn C, Kioussis D, Coles M (2008) Contribution of the neural crest-derived cells in the embryonic and adult thymus. J Immunol 180:3183–3189

Forgacs G (1995) On the possible role of cytoskeletal filamentous networks in intracellular signalling: an approach based on percolation. J Cell Sci 108:2131–2143

Fox NW, Johnstone EM, Ward KE, Schrementi J, Little SP (1997) APP gene promoter constructs are preferentially expressed in CNS and testis of transgenic mice. Biochem Biophys Res Commun 240:759–762

Freeman DA, Rommerts FFG (1996) Regulation of Leydig cell cholesterol transport. In: Payne AH, Hardy MP, Russell LD (eds) The Leydig cell. Cache River, Vienna, 231–239

Frisén J, Johansson CB, Török C, Risling M, Lendahl U (1995) Rapid, widespread, and longlasting induction of nestin contributes to the generation of glial scar tissue after CNS injury. J Cell Biol 131:453–464

Fröjdman K, Pelliniemi LJ, Lendahl U, Virtanen I, Eriksson JE (1997) The intermediate filament protein nestin occurs transiently in differentiating testis of rat and mouse. Differentiation 61:243–249

Frungieri MB, Gonzalez-Calvar SI, Rubio M, Ozu M, Lustig L, Calandra RS (1999) Serotonin in golden hamster testes: testicular levels, immunolocalization and role during sexual development and photoperiodic regression-recrudescence transition. Reprod Neuroendocrinol 69:299–308

Frungieri MB, Urbanski HF, Höhne-Zell B, Mayerhofer A (2000) Neuronal elements in the testis of the rhesus monkey: ontogeny, characterization and relationship to testicular cells. Neuroendocrinology 71:43–50

Frungieri MB, Zitta K, Pignataro OP, Gonzalez-Calvar SI, Calandra RS (2002) Interactions between testicular serotoninergic, catecholaminergic, and corticotropin-releasing hormone systems modulating cAMP and testosterone production in the golden hamster. Neuroendocrinology 76:35–46

Frungieri MB, Mayerhofer A, Zitta K, Pignataro OP, Calandra RS, Gonzalez-Calvar S (2005) Direct effect of melatonin on Syrian hamster testes: melatonin subtype 1a receptors, inhibition of androgen prosuction, and interaction with the local corticotropin-releasing hormone system. Endocrinology 146:1541–1552

Fuchs E (2008) Skin stem cells: rising to the surface. J Cell Biol 180:273–284

Fujimori KE, Kawasaki T, Deguchi T, Yuba S (2008) Characterization of a nervous system-specific promoter for growth-associated protein 43 gene in Medaka (Oryzias latipes). Brain Res 1245:1–15

Fujita T (1989) Present status of paraneuron concept. Arch Histol Cytol 52:1–8

Galli R, Borello U, Gritti A, Minasi MG, Bjornson C, Coletta M, Mora M, De Angilis MG, Fiocco R, Cossu G, Vescovi AL (2000) Skeletal myogenic potential of human and mouse neural stem cells. Nat Neurosci 3:986–991

Galvez BG, Sampoalesi M, Barbuti A, Crespi A, Covarello D, Brunelli S, Dellavalle A, Crippa S, Balconi G, Cuccovillo I, Molla F, Stazewsky L, Latini R, Difrancesco D, Cossu G (2008) Cardiac mesoangioblasts are committed, self-renewable progenitors, associated with small vessels of juvenile mouse ventricle. Cell Death Differ 15:1417–1428

Gaytan F, Aceitero J, Lucena C, Aguilar E, Pinilla L, Garnelo P, Bellido C (1992) Simultaneous proliferation and differentiation of mast cells and Leydig cells in the rat testis. Are common regulatory factors involved? J Androl 13:387–397

Ge R, Hardy MP (2007) Regulation of Leydig cells during pubertal development. In: Payne AH, Hardy MP (eds) Contemporarry endocrinology: the Leydig cell in health and disease. Humana, Totowa, pp 55–70

Ge RS, Shan LX, Hardy MP (1996) Pubertal development of Leydig cells. In: Payne AH, Hardy MP, Russell LD (eds) The Leydig cell. Cache River, Vienna, pp 159–174

Ge RS, Dong Q, Sottas CM, Chen H, Zirkin BR, Hardy MP (2005) Gene expression in rat Leydig cells during development from the progenitor to adult stage: a cluster analysis. Biol Reprod 72:1405–1415

Ge RS, Dong Q, Sottas CM, Papadopoulos V, Zirkin BR, Hardy MP (2006) In search of rat stem Leydig cells: identification, isolation, and lineage-specific development. Proc Natl Acad Sci USA 103:2719–2724

Ge RS, Chen GR, Tanrikut C, Hardy MP (2007) Phthalate ester toxicity in Leydig cells: developmental timing and dosage considerations. Reprod Toxicol 23:366–373

Geigerseder C, Doepner R, Thalhammer A, Frungieri MB, Gamel-Didelon K, Calandra RS, Köhn FM, Mayerhofer A (2003) Evidence for a GABAergic system in rodent and human testis: local GABA production and GABA receptors. Neeuroendocrinology 77:214–232

Geigerseder C, Doepner RFG, Thalhammer A, Krieger A, Mayerhofer A (2004) Stimulation of TM3 Leydig cell proliferation via GABAA receptors: a new role for testicular GABA. Reprod Biol Endocrinol 2:13

Giannessi F, Ruffoli R, Giambelluca MA, Morelli G, Fabris FM (1998) Cytochemical localisation of the NADPH diaphoprase activity in the Leydig cells of the mouse. Histochem Cell Biol 109:241–248

Gibson SJ, Polak JM (1986) Neurochemistry of the spinal cord. In: Polak IM, Van Noorden S (eds) Immunocytochemsitry: modern methods and applications. Wright, Bristol, pp 349–359

Ginsburg M, Snow MH, McLaren A (1990) Primordial germ cells in the mouse embryo during gastrulation. Development 110:521–528

Gnessi L, Emidi A, Farini D, Scarpa S, Modesti A, Ciampani T, Silvestroni L, Spera G (1992) Rat Leydig cells bind platelet-derived growth factor through specific receptors and produce platelet-derived growth factor-like molecules. Endocrinology 130:2219–2224

Gnessi L, Emidi A, Jannini EA, Carosa E, Maroder M, Arizzi M, Ulisse S, Spera G (1995) Testicular development involves the spatiotemporal control of PDGFs and PDGF receptors gene expression and action. J Cell Biol 131:1105–1121

Gnessi L, Basciani S, Mariani S, Arizzi M, Spera G, Wang C, Bondjers C, Karlsson L, Betsholtz C (2000) Leydig cell loss and spermatogenetic arrest in platelet-derived growth factor (PDGF)-A-deficient mice. J. Cell Biol 149:1019–1025

Godin IE, Garcia-Porrero JA, Coutinho A, Dieterlen-Lièvre F, Marcos MAR (1993) Para-aortic splanchnopleura from early mouse embryos contains B1a cell progenitors. Nature 364:67–70

Gondos B (1980) Development and differentiation of the testis and male reproductive tract. In: Steinberger A, Steinberger E (eds) Testicular development structure and function. Raven, New York, pp 3–20

Gritti A, Vescovi AL, Galli R (2002) Adult neural stem cells: plasticity and developmental potential. J Physiol Paris 96:81–90

Grobe JL, Xu D, Sigmund CD (2008) An intracellular rennin-angiotensin system in neurons: fact, hypothesis, or fantasy. Physiol (Bethesda) 23:187–193

Gronthos S, Brohim J, Li W, Fisher LW, Cherman N, Boyde A, DenBeslen P, Robey PG, Shi S (2002) Stem cell properties of human dental pulp stem cells. J Dent Res 81:531–535

Guan K, Wagner S, Unsöld B, Maier LS, Kaiser D, Hemmerlein B, Nayernia K, Engel W, Hasenfuss G (2007) Generation of functional cardiomyocytes from adult mouse spermatogonial stem cells. Circ Res 100:1615–1625

Guldenaar SEF, Pickering BT (1985) Immunocytochemical evidence for the presence of oxytocin in rat testis. Cell Tissue Res 240:485–487

Habert R, Lejeune H, Saez JM (2001) Origin, differentiation and regulation of fetal and adult Leydig cells. Mol Cell Endocrinol 179:47–74

Haider SG (1988) Leydigzellen. Funktionelle Morphologie und Enzymhistochemie bei Ratte und Mensch. Thieme, Stuttgart

Haider SG (2004) Cell biology of Leydig cells in the testis. Int Rev Cytol 233:181–241

Haider SG (2007) Leydig cell steroidogenesis: unmasking the functional importance of mitochondria. Endocrinology 148:2581–2582

Haider SG, Passia D, Overmeyer G (1986) Studies on the fetal and postnatal development of rat Leydig cells employing 3ß-hydroxysteroid dehydrogenase activity. Acta Histochem Suppl 32:197–202

Haider SG, Passia D, Rommert FFG (1990) Histochemical demonstration of 11ß-hydroxysteroid dehydrogenase as a marker for Leydig cell maturation in rat. Acta Histochem Suppl 38:203–207

Haider SG, Laue D, Schwochau G, Hilscher B (1995) Morphological studies on the origin of adult-type Leydig cells in rat testis. Ital J Anat Embryol 100(Suppl 1):535–541

Haider SG, Servos G, Tran N (2007) Structural and histological analysis of Leydig cell steroidogenic function. In: Payne AH, Hardy MP (eds) Contemporarry endocrinology: the Leydig cell in health and disease. Humana, Totowa, pp 33–45

Hall PF, Irby DC, de Kretser DM (1969) Conversion of cholesterol to androgens by rat testes: comparison of interstitial cells and seminiferous tubules. Endocrinology 84:488–496

Hanes FM (1911) The relations of the interstitial cells of Leydig to the production of an internal secretion by the mammalian testis. J Exp Med 13:338–354

Hardy MP, Zirkin BR, Ewing LL (1989) Kinetic studies on the development of the adult population of Leydig cells in testes of the pubertal rat. Endocrinol 124:762–770

Hardy MP, Kelce WR, Klinefelter GR, Ewing LL (1990) Differentiation of Leydig cell precursors in vitro: a role for androgen. Endocrinology 127:488–490

Hart CE, Forstrom JW, Kelly JD, Seifert RA, Smith RA, Ross RA, Murray MJ, Bowen-Pope DF (1988) Two classes of PDGF receptor recognize different isoforms of PDGF. Science 240:1529–1531

Harvey RJ (1875) Über die Zwischensubstanz des Hoden. Centralbl Med Wiss 13(30):497

Hatano O, Takakusu A, Nomura M, Morohashi K (1996) Identical origin of adrenal cortex and gonad revealed by expression profiles of Ad4BP/SF-1. Genes Cells 1:663–671

Hatzopoulos AK, Folkman J, Vasile E, Eiselen GK, Rosenberg RD (1998) Isolation and characterization of endothelial progenitor cells from mouse embryos. Development 125:1457–1468

Hayden MR, Karuparthi PR, Habibi J, Lastra G, Patel K, Wasekar C, Manrique CM, Ozerdem U, Stas S, Sowers JR (2008) Ultrastructure of islet microcirculation, pericytes and islet exocrine interface in the HIP rat model of diabetes. Exp Biol Med 233:1109–1123

He J, Wang Y, Li YL (2007) Fibroblast-like cells derived from gonadal ridges and dorsal mesenteries of human embryos as feeder cells for culture of human embryonic germ cells. J Biomed Sci 14:617–628

Hellström M, Kalén M, Lindahl P, Abramsson A, Betsholtz C (1999) Role of PDGF-B and PDGFR-ß in recruitment of vascular smooth muscle cells and pericytes during embryonic blood vessel formation in the mouse. Development 126:3047–3055

Hellström M, Gerhardt H, Kalen M, Li X, Eriksson U, Wolburg H, Betsholtz C (2001) Lack of pericytes leads to endothelial hyperplasia and abnormal vascular morphogenesis. J Cell Biol 153:543–553

Henle J (1866) Handbuch der Eingeweidelehre des Menschen. Handbuch der systematischen Anatomie des Menschen, vol 2. Vieweg, Braunschweig, p 538

Herzog EL, Chai L, Krause DS (2003) Plasticity of marrow-derived stem cells. Blood 102:3483–3493

Hess DC, Abe T, Hill WD, Studdard AM, Carothers J, Masuya M, Fleming PA, Drake CJ, Ogawa M (2004) Hematopoietic origin of microglial and perivascular cells in brain. Exp Neurol 186:134–144

Hirschi KK, D'Amore PA (1996) Pericytes in the microvasculature. Cardiovasc Res 32:687–698

Hirschi KK, Majesky MW (2004) Smooth muscle stem cells. Anat Rec Part A Discov Mol Cell Evol Biol 276A:22–33

Hirschi KK, Rohovsky SA, Beck LH, Smith SR, D'Amore PA (1999) Endothelial cells modulate the proliferation of mural cell precursors via platelet-derived growth factor-BB and heterotypic cell contact. Circ Res 84:298–305

Hofmeister H (1872) Untersuchungen über die Zwischensubstanz im Hoden der Säugetiere. Sitzungsber MathNaturwiss Cl Kais Akad Wiss Wien 65(3):77–100

Holash JA, Harik SI, Perry G, Stewart PA (1993) Barrier properties of testis microvessels. Proc Natl Acad Sci USA 90:11069–11073

Holmgren L, Glaser A, Pfeifer-Ohlson S, Ohlson R (1991) Angiogenesis during human extraembryonic development involves the spatiotemporal control of PDGF ligand and receptor gene expression. Development 113:749–754

Holstein AF, Davidoff MS (1997) Organization of the intertubular tissue of the human testis. In: PM Motta (ed.) Recent advances in microscopy of cells, tissues and organs. Delfino, Rome, pp 569–577

Holstein AF, Roosen-Runge EC (1981) Atlas of human spermatogenesis. Grosse,Berlin, pp 1–224

Holstein AF, Wartenberg H, Vossmeyer J (1971) Zur Cytologie der pränatalen Gonadenentwicklung beim Menschen. III Die Entwicklung der Leydigzellen im Hoden von Embryonen und Feten. Z Anal Entwickl Gesch 135:43–66

Holstein AF, Roosen-Rungc EC, Schirren C (1988) Illustrated pathology of human spermatogenesis. Grosse, Berlin, pp 1–278

Holstein AF, Maekawa M, Nagano T, Davidoff MS (1996) Myofibroblasts of the lamina propria of the human seminiferous tubules are dynamic structures of heterogeneous phenotype. Arch Histol Cytol 59:109–125

Hökfelt T, Lundberg JM, Schulzberg M, Jahansson O, Ljundahl A, Rehfeld J (1980) Coexistence of peptides and putative transmitters in neurons. In: Costa E, Trabucci M (eds) Neural peptides and neural communication. Raven, New York, pp 1–23

Hoofnagle MH, Wamhoff BR, Owens GK (2004) Lost of transdifferentiation. J Clin Invest 113:1249–1251

Horwitz EM, Le Blanc K, Dominici M, Mueller I, Slaper-Cortenbach I, Marani FC, Deans RJ, Krause DS, Keating A, The International Society for Cellular Therapy (2005) Clarification of nomenclature for MSC: the International Society for Cellular Therapy position statement. Cytotherapy 7:393–395

Howson KM, Aplin AC, Gelati M, Alessandri G, Parati EA, Nicosia RF (2005) The postnatal rat aorta contains pericyte progenitor cells that form spheroidal colonies in suspension culture. Am J Physiol Cell Physiol 289:C1396–C1407

Hu JH, Zhang JF, Ma YH, Jiang J, Yang N, Li XB, Yu Chi ZC, Fei J, Guo LH (2004) Impaired reproduction in transgenic mice overexpressing γ-aminobutyric acid transporter I (GAT1). Cell Res 14:54–59

Hu Y, Zhang Z, Torsney E, Afzal AR, Davison F, Metzler B, Xu Q (2004) Abundant progenitor cells in the adventitia contribute to atherosclerosis of vein grafts in ApoE-deficient mice. J Clin Invest 113:1258–1265

Huhtaniemi I, Pelliniemi LJ (1992) Fetal Leydig cells: cellular origin, morphology, life span, and special functional features. Proc Soc Exp Biol Med 201:125–140

Huhtaniemi I, Toppari J (1995) Endocrine, paracrine and autocrine regulation of testicular steroidogenesis. In: Mukhopadhyay AK, Raizada MK (eds) Tissue renin-angiotensin systems. Current concepts of local regulators in reproductive and endocrine organs. Plenum, New York, pp 33–54

Hunziker E, Stein M (2000) Nestin-expressing cells in the pancreatic islets of Langerhans. Biochem Biophys Res Commun 29:116–119

Hutson JC (1990) Changes in the concentration and size of testicular macrophages during development. Biol Reprod 43:885–890

Ihrie RA, Alvarez-Builla A (2008) Cells in the astroglial lineage are neural stem cells. Cell Tissue Res 331:179–191

Ilancheran S, Michalska A, Peh G, Wallace EM, Pera M, Manuelpillai U (2007) Stem cells derived from human fetal membranes display multilineage differentiation potential. Biol Reprod 77:577–588

Ishisaki A, Hayashi H, Li A-J, Imamura T (2003) Human umbilical vein endothelium-derived cells retain potential to differentiate into smooth muscle-like cells. J Biol Chem 278:1303–1309

Iskaros J, Pickard M, Evans I, Sinha A, Hardiman P, Ekins R (2000) Thyroid hormone receptor gene expression in first trimester human fetal brain. J Clin Endocrinol Metab 65:2620–2623

Ito S, Komatsu K, Yajima Y, Hirayama A (2008) Renin-angiotensin system in the brain as a new target of antihypertensive therapy. Hypertens Res 31:1487–1488

Ivell R, Furuja K, Brackmann B, Dawood Y, Khan-Dawood F (1990) Expression of oxytocin and vasopressin genes in human and baboon gonadal tissues. Endocrinology 127:2990–2996

Jackson AE, O'Leary PC, Ayers MM, de Kretser DM (1986) The effects of ethylene dimethane sulphonate (EDS) on rat Leydig cells: evidence to support a connective tissue origin of Leydig cells. Biol Reprod 35:425–437

Jackson CM, Jackson H (1984) Comparative protective actions of gonadotrophins and testosterone against the antispermatogenic action of ethane dimethanesulphonate. J Reprod Fertil 71:393–401

Jackson KA, Mi T, Goodell MA (1999) Hematopoietic potential of stem cells isolated from murine skeletal muscle. Proc Natl Acad Sci USA 96:14482–14486

Jackson KA, Majka SM, Wang H, Pocius J, Hartley CJ, Majeski MW, Entman ML, Michael LH, Hirschi KK, Goodell MA (2001) Regeneration of ischemic cardiac muscle and vascular endothelium by adult stem cells. J Clin Invest 107:1395–1402

Jackson NC, Jackson H, Shanks JH, Dixon JS, Lendon RG (1986) Study using in-vivo binding of 125I-labelled hCG, light and electron microscopy of the repupolation or rat Leydig cells after destruction due to administration of ethylene-1,2-dimethanesulphonate. J Reprod Fert 76:1–10

Jacobson A (1879) Zur pathologischen Histologie der traumatischen Hodenentzündung. Virchows Arch Pathol Anat Physiol Klin Med 75:349–398

Jaffredo T, Gautier R, Eichmann A, Dieterlen-Lièvre F (1998) Intraaortic hemopoietic cells are derived from endothelial cells during ontogeny. Development 125:4575–4583

Jeanes A, Wilhelm D, Wilson MJ, Bowles J, McClive PJ, Sinclair AH, Koopman P (2005) Evaluation of candidate markers for peritubular myoid cell lineage in the developing mouse testis. Reproduction 130:509–516

Jeays-Ward K, Hoyle C, Brennan J, Dandonneau M, Alldus G, Capel B, Swain A (2003) Endothelial and steroidogenic cell migration are regulated by WNT4 in the developing mammalian gonad. Development 130:3663–3670

Jeffs B, Meeks JJ, Ito M, Martinson FA, Matzuk MM, Jameson JL, Russell LD (2001) Blockage of the rete testis and efferent ductules by ectopic Sertoli and Leydig cells causes infertility in Dax-1-deficient mice. Endocrinology 142:4486–4495

Jégou B, Pineau C (1995) Current aspects of autocrine and paracrine regulation of spermatogenesis. In: Mukhopadhyay AK, Raizada MK (eds) Tissue rennin-angiotensin systems. Current concepts of local regulators in reproductive and endocrine organs. Plenum, New York, pp 67–86

Jiang Y, Vaessen B, Lenvik T, Blackstad M, Reyes M, Verfaillie CM (2002) Multipotent progenitor cells can be isolated from postnatal murine bone marrow, muscle, and brain. Exp Hematol 30:896–904

Jiang Y, Henderson D, Blackstad M, Chen A, Miller RF, Verfaillie CM (2003) Neuroectodermal differentiation from mouse multipotent adult progenitor cells. Proc Natl Acad Sci USA 100:11854–11860

Jiang S, Walker L, Afentoulis DA, Jauron-Mills L, Corless CL, Fleming WH (2004) Transplanted human bone marrow contributes to vascular endothelium. Proc Natl Acad Sci USA 101:16891–16896

Jin K, Zhu Y, Sun Y, Mao XO, Xie L, Greenberg DA (2002) Vascular endothelial growth factor (VEGF) stimulates neurogenesis in vitro and in vivo. Proc Natl Acad Sci USA 99:11946–11950

Jin S, Hansson EM, Tikka S, Lanner F, Sahlgren C, Farnebo F, Baumann M, Kalimo H, Lendahl U (2008) Notch signaling regulates platelet-derived growth factor receptor-ß expression in vascular smooth muscle cells. Circ Res 102:1483–1491

Jorens PG, Matthys KE, Bult H (1995) Modulation of nitric oxide synthase activity in macrophages. Mediat Inflamm 4:75–89

Joseph NM, Mukouyama Y-s, Mosher JT, Jaegle M, Crone SA, Dormand E-L, Lee K-F, Meijer D, Anderson DJ, Morrison SJ (2004) Neural crest stem cells undergo multilineage differentiation in developing peripheral nerves to generate endoneurial fibroblasts in addition to Schwann cells. Development 131:5599–5612

Josephson R, Müller T, Pickel J, Reynolds K, Turner PA, Zimmer A, McKay RDG (1998) POU transcription factors control expression of CNS stem cell-specific genes. Development 125:3087–3100

Kajahn J, Gorjup E, Tiede S, von Briesen H, Paus R, Kruse C, Danner S (2008) Skin-derived adult stem cells surprisingly share many features with human pancreatic stem cells. Eur J Cell Biol 87:39–46

Kajstura J, Urbanek K, Rota M, Bearzi C, Hosoda T, Bolli R, Anversa P, Leri A (2008) Cardiac stem cells and myocardial disease. J Mol Cell Cardiol 45:505–513

Kale S, Karihaloo A, Clark PR, Kashgarian M, Krause DS, Cantley LG (2003) Bone marrow stem cells contribute to repair of the ischemically injured renal tubule. J Clin Invest 112:42–49

Kamath SG, Chen N, Enkemann SA, Sanchez-Ramos J (2005) Transcriptional profile of NeuroD expression in a human fetal astroglial cell line. Gene Expr 12:123–136

Kanatsu-Shinohara M, Inoue K, Lee J, Yoshimoto M, Ogonuki N, Miki H, Baba S, Kato T, Kazuki Y, Toyokuni S, Toyoshima M, Niwa O, Oshimura M, Heike T, Nakahata T, Ishino F, Ogura A, Shinohara T (2004) Generation of pluripotent stem cells from neonatal mouse testis. Cell 119:1001–1012

Kanchev LN, Konakchieva R, Angelova PA, Davidoff MS (1995) Substance P modulating effect on the binding capacity of hamster Leydig cell LH receptors. Life Sci 56:1631–1637

Kanzaki M, Fujisawa M, Okuda Y, Okada H, Arikawa S, Kamidono S (1996) Expression and regulation of neuropeptide Y messenger ribonucleic acid in cultured immature rat Leydig and Sertoli cells. Endocrinology 137:1249–1257

Karl J, Capel B (1998) Sertoli cells of the mouse testis originate from coelomic epithelium. Dev Biol 203:323–333

Kermani P, Rafii D, Jin DK, Whitlock P, Schaffer W, Chiang A, Vincent L, Friedrich M, Shido K, Hackett NR, Crystal RG, Rafii S, Hempstead BL (2005) Neurotrophins promote revascularization by local recruitment of TrkB+ endothelial cells and systemic mobilization of hematopoietic progenitors. J Clin Invest 115:653–663

Kerr JB, de Kretser DM (1981) The cytology of the human testis. In: Burger H, de Kretser DM (eds) Comprehensive endocrinology: the testis. Raven, New York, pp 141–169

Kerr JB, Donachie K (1986) Regeneration of Leydig cells in unilaterally cryptorchid rats: evidence for stimulation by local testicular factors. Cell Tissue Res 245:649–655

Kerr JB, Knell CM (1988) The fate of fetal Leydig cells during the development of the fetal and postnatal rat testis. Development 103:535–544

Kerr JB, Sharpe RM (1985) Stimulatory effect of follicle-stimulating hormone on rat Leydig cells. A morphometric and ultrastructural study. Cell Tissue Res 239:405–415

Kerr JB, Donachie K, Rommerts FFG (1985) Selective destruction and regeneration of rat Leydig cells in vivo. A new method for the study of seminiferous tubular-interstitial tissue interaction. Cell Tissue Res 242:145–156

Kerr JB, Bartlett JMS, Donachie K (1986) Acute response of testicular interstitial tissue in rats to the cytotoxic drug ethane dimethanesulphonate. An ultrastructural and hormonal study. Cell Tissue Res 243:405–414

Kerr JB, Knell CM, Abbott M, Donachie K (1987a) Ultrastructural analysis of the effect of ethane dimethanesulphoante on the testis of the rat, guinea pig, hamster and mouse. Cell Tissue Res 249:451–457

Kerr JB, Bartlett JMS, Donachie K, Sharpe RM (1987b) Origin of regenerating Leydig cells in the testis of the adult rat. An ultrastructural, morphometric and hormonal assay study. Cell Tissue Res 249:367–377

Kerr JB, Risbridger GP, Knell CM (1988) Stimulation of interstitial cell growth after selective destruction of foetal Leydig cells in the testis of postnatal rats. Cell Tissue Res 252:89–98

Kerr JB, Millar M, Maddocks S, Sharpe RM (1993) Stage-dependent changes in spermatogenesis and Sertoli cells in relation to the onset of spermatogenesis failure following withdrawal of testosterone. Anat Rec 235:547–559

Keshet E, Lyman SD, Williams DE, Anderson DM, Jenkins NA, Copeland NG, Parada LF (1991) Embryonic RNA expression patterns of the c-kit receptor and cognate ligand suggest multiple functional roles in mouse development. EMBO J 10:2425–2435

Khurana ML, Pandey KN (1993) Receptor-mediated stimulatory effect of atrial natriuretic factor, brain natriuretic peptide, and C-type natriuretic peptide on testosterone production in purified mouse Leydig cells: activation of cholesterol side-chain cleavage enzyme. Endocrinology 133:2141–2149

Kiel MJ, Morrison SJ (2006) Maintaining hematopoietic stem cells in the vascular niche. Immunity 25:862–864

Kim H, Li Q, Hempstead BL, Madri JA (2004) Paracrine and autocrine functions of brain-derived neurotrophic factor (BDNF) and nerve growth factor (NGF) in brain-derived endothelial cells. J Biol Chem 279:3538–3546

Kim Y, Capel B (2006) Balancing the bipotential gonad between alternative organ fates: a new perspective on an old problem. Dev Dyn 235:2292–2300

Kim Y, Kobayashi A, Sekido R, DiNapoli L, Brennan J, Chaboissier M-C, Poulat F, Behringer RR, Lovell-Badge R, Capel B (2006) Fgf9 and Wnt4 act as antagonistic signals to regulate mammalian sex determination. PLoS Biol 4(6):e187.doi:10.1371/journal.pbio.0040187

Klein T, Ling Z, Heimberg H, Madsen OD, Heller RS, Serup P (2003) Nestin is expressed in vascular endothelial cells in the adult human pancreas. J Histochem Cytochem 5:697–706

Klinefelter GR, Laskey JW, Roberts NL (1991) In vitro/in vivo effects of ethane dimethanesulfonate on Leydig cells of adult rats. Toxicol Appl Pharmacol 107:460–471

Klinefelter G, Kelce WR (1996) Leydig cell responsiveness to hormonal and non-hormonal factors in vivo and in vitro. In: Payne AH, Hardy MP, Russell LD (eds) The Leydig cell. Cache River, Vienna, 535–553

Kobayashi A, Chang H, Chaboissier M-C, Schedl A, Behringer RR (2005) Sox9 in testis development. Ann N Y Acad Sci 1061:9–17

Kobayashi H, DeBusk LM, Babichev YO, Dumont DJ, Lin PC (2006) Hepatocyte growth factor mediates angiopoietin-induced smooth muscle cell recruitment. Blood 108:1260–1266

Koeva YA, Bakalska MV, Atanassova NN, Davidoff MS (2008a) INSLF3-LGR8 ligand-receptor system in testes of mature rats after exposure to ethane dimethanesulphonate (short communication). Folia Med 50:37–42

Koeva YA, Bakalska MV, Atanassova NN, Davidoff MS (2008b) c-erbAalpha and c-erbAbeta in the Leydig cell repopulation by ethane-1,2-dimethanesulphonate model of mature rats. Folia Med (Plovdiv) 50:53–57

Koike S, Noumura T (1993) Immunohistochemical localizations of TGF-ß in the developing rat gonads. Zool Sci 10:671–677

Kölliker A (1854) Mikroskopische Anatomie der Gewebelehre des Menschen, vol 2. Engelmann, Leipzig

Koopman P (2005) Sex determination: a tale of two Sox genes. Trends Genet 21:367–370

Koopman P, Münsterberg A, Capel B, Vivian N, Lovell-Badge R (1990) Expression of a candidate sex-determining gene during mouse testis development. Nature 348:450–452

Koopman P, Gubbay J, Vivian N, Goodfellow P, Lovell-Badge R (1991) Male development of chromosomally female mice transgenic for Sry. Nature 351:117–121

Kopp HG, Hooper AT, Shmelkov SV, Rafii S (2007) Beta-galactosidase staining on bone marrow. The osteoclast pitfall. Histol Histopathol 22:971–976

Kopp J, Collin O, Villar M, Mullins D, Bergh A, Hökfelt T (2008) Regulation of neuropeptide Y Y1 receptors by testosterone in vascular smooth muscle cells in rat testis. Neuroendocrinology 88:216–226

Korn J, Christ B, Kurz H (2002) Neuroectodermal origin of brain pericytes and vascular smooth muscle cells. J Comp Neurol 442:78–88

Kostic TS, Andric SA, Maric D, Stojilkovic SS, Kovacevic R (1999) Involvement of inducible nitric oxide synthase in stress-impaired testicular steroidogenesis. J Endocrinol 163:409–416

Krause DS, Theise ND, Collector MI, Henegariu O, Hwang S, Gardner R, Neutzel S, Sharkis SJ (2001) Multi-organ, multi-lineage engraftment by a single bone marrow-derived stem cell. Cell 105:369–377

Kruger GM, Mosher JT, Bixby S, Joseph N, Iwashita T, Morrison SJ (2002) Neural crest stem cells persist in the adult gut but undergo changes in self-renewal, neuronal subtype potential, and factor responsiveness. Neuron 35:657–669

Kruse C, Birth M, Rohwedel J, Assmuth K, Goepel A, Wedel T (2004) Pluripotency of adult stem cells derived from human and rat pancreas. Appl Phys A 79:1617–1624

Kruse C, Bodó E, Petschnik AE, Danner S, Tiede S, Paus R (2006a) Towards the development of a pragmatic technique for isolating and differentiating nestin-positive cells from human scalp skin into neuronal and glial cells populations: generating neurons from human skin ?Exp Dermatol 15:794–800

Kruse C, Kajan J, Petschnik AE, Maaß A, Klink E, Rapoport DH, Wedel T (2006b) Adult pancreatic stem/progenitor cells spontaneously differentiate in vitro into multiple cell lineages and form teratoma-like structures. Ann Anat 188:503–517

Kuang S, Kuroda K, Le Grand F, Rudnicki MA (2007) Assymetric self-renewal and commitment of satelite stem cells in muscle. Cell 129:999–1010

Kubo H, Alitalo K (2003) The bloody fate of endothelial stem cells. Genes Dev 17:322–329

Kubota H, Avarbock MR, Brinster RL (2003) Spermatogonial stem cells share some, but not all, phenotypic and functional characteristics with other stem cells. Proc Natl Acad Sci USA 100:6487–6492

Kucia M, Machalinski B, Ratajczak MZ (2006a) The developmental deposition of epiblast/germ cell-line derived cells in various organs as a hypothetical explanation of stem cell plasticity? Acta Neurobiol Exp (Waes) 66:331–341

Kucia M, Zhang YP, Reca R, Wysoczynski M, Machalinski B, Majka M, Ildstad ST, Ratajczak J, Shields CB, Ratajczak MZ (2006b) Cells enriched in markers of neural tissue-committed stem cells reside in the bone marrow and are mobilized into the peripheral blood following stroke. Leukemia 20:18–28

Kucia M, Suba-Surma E, Wysoczynski M, Dobrowolska H, Reca R, Ratajczak J, Ratajczak MZ (2006d) Physiological and pathological consequences of identification of very small embryonic like (VSEL) stem cells in adult bone marrow. J Physiol Pharmacol 57(Suppl 5):5–18

Kucia M, Wu W, Ratajczak MZ (2007) Bone marrow-derived very small embryonic-like stem cells: their developmental origin and biological significance. Dev Dyn 236:3309-3320

Kuhn HG, Palmer TD, Fuchs E (2001) Adult neurogenesis: a compensatory mechanism for neuronal damage. Eur Arch Psychiatry Clin Neurosci 251:152–158

Kukucka MA, Misra HP (1993) The antioxidant defence system of isolated guinea pig Leydig cells. Mol Cell Biochem 126:1–7

Kuopio T, Pelliniemi LJ (1989) Patchy basement membranes of rat Leydig cells shown by ultrastructural immunolabeling. Cell Tissue Res 256:45–51

Kuopio T, Paranko J, Pelliniemi LJ (1989a) Basement membrane and epithelial features of fetal-type Leydig cells in rat and human testis. Differentiation 40:198–206

Kuopio T, Pelliniemi LJ, Huhtaniemi I (1989b) Rapid Leydig cell proliferation and LH receptor replenishment after single injection of human chorionic gonadotropin in the neonatal rat testis. Biol Reprod 40:135–143

Kuopio T, Tapanainen J, Pelliniemi LJ, Huhtaniemi I (1989c) Developmental stages of fetal-type Leydig cells in prepubertal rats. Development 107:213–220

Kuznetsov SA, Mankani MH, Leet AI, Ziran N, Gronthos S, Robey PG (2007) Circulating connective tissue precursors: extreme rarity in humans and chondrogenic potential in guinea pigs. Stem Cells 25:1830–1839

LaBarge MA, Blau HM (2002) Biological progression from adult bone marrow to mononuclear muscle stem cell to multinucleate muscle fiber in response to injury. Cell 111:589–601

Lagasse E, Connors H, Al-Dhalimy, Reitsma M, Dohse M, Osborne L, Wang X, Finegold M, Weissman IL, Grompe M (2000) Purified hematopoietic stem cells can differentiate into hepatocytes in vivo. Nat Med 6:1229–1234

Lai EC (2004) Notch signalling: control of cell communication and cell fate. Development 131:965–973

Lammert E, Cleaver O, Melton D (2001) Induction of pancreatic differentiation by signals from blood vessels. Science 294:564–567

Lardon J, Rooman I, Bowens L (2002) Nestin expression in pancreatic stellate cells and angiogenic endothelial cells. Histochem Cell Biol 117:535–540

Lauke H, Behrens K, Holstein AF (1989) Leydig cell mitoses in human testes bearing early germ cell tumors. Cell Tissue Res 255:475–479

Lechner A, Leech CA, Abraham EJ, Nolan AL, Habner JF (2002) Nestin-positive progenitor cells derived from adult human pancreatic islets of Langerhans contain side population (SP) cells defined by expression of the ABCG2 (BCRP1) ATP-binding cassette transporter. Biochem Biophys Res Commun 293:670–674

LeCouter J, Lin R, Tejada M, Frantz G, Peale F, Hillan KJ, Ferrara N (2003) The endocrine-gland-derived VEGF homologue Bv8 promotes angiogenesis in the testis: localization of Bv8 receptors to endothelial cells. Proc Natl Acad Sci USA 100:2685–2690

LeCouter J, Zlot C, Tejada M, Peale F, Ferrara N (2004) Bv8 and endocrine gland-derived vascular endothelial growth factor stimulate hematopoiesis and hematopoietic cell mobilization. Proc Natl Acad Sci USA 101:16813–16818

Le Douarin NM, Creuzet S, Couly G, Dupin E (2004) Neural crest cell plasticity and its limits. Development 131:4637–4650

Le Douarin NM, Brito JM, Creuzet S (2007) Role of neural crest in face and brain development. Brain Res Rev 55:237–242

Le Douarin NM, Calloni GW, Dupin E (2008) The stem cells of the neural crest. Cell Cycle 7:1013–1019

Lee JS, Semela D, Iredale J, Shah VH (2007) Sinusoidal remodeling and angiogenesis: a new function for the liver-specific pericyte. Hepathology 45:817–825

Lejeune H, Habert R, Saez JM (1998) Origin, proliferation and differentiation of Leydig cells. J Mol Endocrinol 20:1–25

Lemkine GF, Raji A, Alfama G, Turque N, Hassani Z, Alegria-Prévot O, Samarut J, Levi G, Demeneix BA (2005) Adult neural stem cell cycling in vivo requires thyroid hormone and its alpha receptor. FASEB J 19:863–865

Leydig F (1850) Zur Anatomie der männlichen Geschlechtsorgane und Analdrüsen der Säugetiere. Z Wiss Zool 2:1–57

Li A, Pouliot N, Redvers R, Kaur P (2004) Extensive tissue-regenerative capacity of neonatal human keratinocyte stem cells and their progeny. J Clin Invest 113:390–400

Li L, Mignone J, Yang M, Matic M, Penman S, Enikolopov G, Hoffman RM (2003) Nestin expression in hair follicle sheath progenitor cells. Proc Natl Acad Sci USA 100:9958–9961

Lim DA, Alvarez-Buylla A (1999) Interaction between astrocytes and adult subventricular zone precursors stimulates neurogenesis. Proc Natl Acad Sci USA 96:7526–7531

Lin L-FH, Doherty DH, Lile JD Bektesh S, Collins F (1993) GDNF: a glial cell-derived neurotrophic factor for midbrain dopaminergic neurons. Science 260:1130–1132

Lin G, Garcia M, Ning H, Banie L, Guo Y-L, Lue TF, Lin C-S (2008) Defining stem and progenitor cells within adipose tissue. Stem Cells Dev 17:1–12

Lindahl P, Karlsson L, Hellström M, Gebre-Medhin S, Willetts K, Heath JK, Betsholtz C (1997a) Alveogenesis failure in PDGF-A-deficient mice is coupled to lack of distal spreading of alveolar smooth muscle cell progenitors during lung development. Development 124:3943–3953

Lindahl P, Johansson BR, Leveen P, Betsholtz C (1997b) Pericyte loss and microaneurism formation in PDGF-B-deficient mice. Science 277:242–245

Lindblom P, Gerhardt H, Liebner S, Abramsson A, Enge M, Hellström M, Bäckström G, Fredricsson S, Landegren U, Nyström HC, Bergström G, Dejana E, Östman A, Lindahl P, Betsholtz C (2003) Endothelial PDGF-B retention is required for proper investment of pericytes in the microvessel wall. Genes Dev 17:1835–1840

Lindskog H, Athley E, Larsson E, Lundin S, Hellström S, Lindahl P (2006) New insights to vascular smooth muscle cell and pericyte differentiation of mouse embryonic stem cells in vitro. Arterioscler Thromb Vasc Biol 26:1457–1464

Lissbrant E, Löfmark U, Collin O, Bergh A (1997) Is nitric oxide involved in the regulation of the rat testicular vasculature? Biol Reprod 56:1221–1227

Liu H, Gronthos S, Shi S (2006) Dental pulp stem cells. Methods Enzymol 419:99–113

Liu K, Wang Z, Wang H, Zhang Y (2002) Nestin expression and proliferation of ependymal cells in adult rat spinal cord after injury. Chin Med J 115:339–341

Lo KC, Lei Z, Rao CV, Beck J, Lamb DJ (2004) De novo testosterone production in luteinizing hormone receptor knockout mice after transplantation of Leydig stem cells. Endocrinology 145:4011–4015

Lobo MVT, Arenas MI, Alonso FJM, Gomez G, Bazán E, Paino C, Fernández E, Fraile B, Paniagua R, Moyano A, Caso E (2004) Nestin, a neuroectodermal stem cell marker molecule, is expressed in Leydig cells of the human testis and some specific cell types from human testicular tumours. Cell Tissue Res 316:369–376

Lording DW, de Kretser DM (1972) Comparative ultrastructural and histochemical studies of the interstitial cells of the rat testis during fetal and postnatal development. J Reprod Fertil 29:261–269

Lothian C, Lendahl U (1997) An evolutionarily conserved region in the second intron of the human nestin gene directs gene expression to CNS progenitor cells and to early neural crest cells. Eur J Neurosci 9:452–462

Louissaint A Jr, Rao S, Leventhal C, Goldman SA (2002) Coordinated interaction of neurogenesis and angiogenesis in the adult songbird brain. Neuron 34:945–960

Lovell-Badge R, Robertson E (1990) XY female mice resulting from heritable mutation in the primary testis-determining gene, Tdy. Development 109:635–646

Lue YH, Ekkila K, Liu PY, Ma K, Wang C, Hikim AS, Swerdloff RS (2007) Fate of bone marrow stem cells transplanted into the testis. Potential implication for men with testiuclar failure. Am J Pathol 170:899–908

Lukyanenko Y, Chen J-J, Hutson JC (2001) Production of 25-hydroxycholesterol by testicular macrophages and ist effects on leydig cells. Biol Reprod 64:790–796

Luo X, Ikeda Y, Parker KL (1994) A cell-specific nuclear receptor is essential for adrenal and gonadal development and sexual differentiation. Cell 77:481–490

Majesky MW (2007) Developmental basis of vascular smooth muscle diversity. Arterioscler Thromb Vasc Biol 27:1248–1258

Majdic G, Saunders PTK, Teerds KJ (1998) Immunoexpression of the steroidogenic enzymes 3-beta hydroxysteroid dehydrogenase and 17α-hydroxylase, C17,20 lyase and the receptor for luteinizing hormone (LH) in the fetal rat testis suggests that the onset of Leydig cell steroid production is independent of LH action. Biol Reprod 58:520–525

Makabe S, Naguro T, Heyn R, Motta PM (1995) Ultrastructure of human Leydig cells at early gonadal embryogenesis. Ital J Anat Embryol 100(Suppl 1):525–533

Mancini RE, Vilar O, Lavieri JC, Andrada JA, Heinrich JJ (1963) Development of Leydig cells in the normal human testis: a cytological, cytochemical and quantitative study. Am J Anat 112:203–214

Mancino MG, Carpino G, Onori P, Franchitto A, Alvaro D, Gaudio E (2007) Hepatic "stem" cells: state of the art. Ital J Anat Embryol 112:93–109

Mariani S, Basciani S, Arizzi M, Spera G, Gnessi L (2002) PDGF and the testis. Trends Endocrinol Metab 13:11–17

Marcus AJ, Woodbury D (2008) Fetal stem cells from extra-embryonic tissues: do not discard. J Cell Mol Med 12:730–742

Margioris AN, Liotta AS, Vaudry H, Bardin CW, Krieger DT (1983) Characterization of immunoreactive proopiomelanocortin-related peptides in rat testes. Endocrinology 113:663–671

Martens TP, See F, Schuster MD, Sondermaijer HP, Hefti MM, Zannettino A, Gronthos S, Seki T, Itescu S (2006) Mesenchymal lineage precursor cells induce vascular network formation in ischemic myocardium. Nat Clin Pract Cardiovasc Med 3(Suppl 1):S18–S22

Martineau J, Nordqvist K, Tilmann C, Lovell-Badge R, Capel B (1997) Male-specific cell migration into the developing gonad. Curr Biol 7:958–968

Masuya M, Drake CJ, Fleming PA, Reilly CM, Zeng H, Hill WD, Martin-Studdard A, Hess DC, Ogawa M (2003) Hematopoietic origin of glomerular mesangial cells. Blood 101:2215–2218

Matsui Y, Zsebo KM, Hogan BL (1990) Embryonic expression of a hematopoietic growth factor encoded by the S1 locus and the ligand for c-kit. Nature 347:667–669

Matsuoka S, Tsuji K, Hisakawa H, Xu M-j, Ebihara Y, Ishi T, Sugiyama D, Manabe A, Tanaka R, Ikeda Y, Asano S, Nakahata T (2001) Generation of definitive hematopoietic stem cells from murine early yolk sac and paraaortic splanchnopleures by aorta-gonad-mesonephros region-derived stromal cells. Blood 98:6–12

Maunoury R, Portier MM, Léonard N, McCormick D (1991) Glial fibrillary acidic protein immunoreactivity in adrenocortical and Leydig cells of the Syrian golden hamster (Mesocricetus auratus). J Neuroimmunol 35:119–129

Mayerhofer A (1996) Leydig cell regulation by catecholamines and neuroendocrine messengers. In: Payne AH, Hardy MP, Russell LD (eds) The Leydig cell. Cache River, Vienna, pp 407–417

Mayerhofer A (2007) Neuronal signalling molecules and Leydig cells. In: Payne AH, Hardy MP (eds) Contemporarry endocrinology: the Leydig cell in health and disease. Humana, Totowa, pp 291–304

Mayerhofer A, Frungieri MB, Fritz S, Bulling A, Jessberger B, Vogt H-J (1999) Evidence for catecholamineergic, neuronlike cells in the adult human testis: changes associated with testicular pathologies. J Androl 20:341–347

Mayerhofer A, Seidl K, Lahr G, Bitter-Suermann D, Christoph A, Barthels D, Wille W, Gratzl M (1992) Leydig cells express neural cell adhesion molecules in vivo and in vitro. Biol Reprod 47:656–664

Mayerhofer A, Lahr G, Seidl K, Eusterschulte B, Christoph A, Gratzl M (1996) The neural cell adhesion molecule (NCAM) provides clues to the development of testicular Leydig cells. J Androl 17:223–230

McKay R (1997) Stem cells in the central nervous system. Science 276:66–71

McLaren A (1991) Development of the mammalian gonad: the fate of the supporting lineage. Bioessays 13:151–156

McLaren A (1998) Gonad development: assembling the mammalian testis. Curr Biol 8:R175–R177

McLaren A (2000) Germ and somatic cell lineages in the developing gonad. Mol Cell Endocrinol 163:3–9

McLaren A (2003) Primordial germ cells in the mouse. Dev Biol 262:1–15

Medvinsky AL, Samoylina NL, Muller AM, Dzierzak EA (1993) An early pre-liver intraembryonic source of CFU-S in the developing mouse. Nature 364:64–67

Mendis-Handagama SMLC, Risbridger GP, de Kretser DM (1987) Morphometric analysis of the components of the neonatal and the adult rat testis interstitium. Int J Androl 10:525–534

Mendis-Handagama SMLC, Ariyaratne HB (2001) Differentiation of the adult Leydig cell population in the postnatal testis. Biol Reprod 65:660–671

Mendis-Handagama SM, Ariyaratne HB (2008) Effects of hypothyroidism on anti-mullerian hormone expression in the prepubertal rat testis. Histol Histopathol 23:151–156

Menthena A, Deb N, Oertel M, Grozdanov PN, Sandhu J, Shah S, Guha C, Shafritz DA, Dabeva MD (2004) Bone marrow progenitors are not the source of expanding oval cells in injected liver. Stem Cells 22:1049–1061

Merchant-Larios H, Moreno-Mendoza N (1998) Mesonephric stromal cells differentiate into Leydig cells in the mouse fetal testis. Exp Cell Res 244:230–238

Merchant-Larios H, Moreno-Mendoza N, Buehr M (1993) The role of the mesonephros in cell differentiation and morphogenesis of the mouse testis. Int J Dev Biol 37:407–415

Mercier F, Kitasako JT, Hatton GI (2002) Anatomy of the brain neurogenic zones revisited: fractones and the fibroblast/macrophage network. J Comp Neurol 451:170–188

Messam CA, Hou J, Major EO (2000) Coexpression of nestin in neural and glial cells in the developing human CNS defined by a human-specific anti-nestin antibody. Exp Neurol 161:585–596

Meyrick B, Reid L (1978) The effect of continued hypoxia on rat pulmonary arterial circulation. Lab Invest 38:188–200

Meyrick B, Reid L (1979) Ultrastructural features of the distended pulmonary arteries of the neonatal rat. Anat Rec 193:71–98

Miao J, Chan K-W, Chen GG, Chun S-Y, Xia N-S, Chan JYH, Panesar NS (2005) Blocking BRE expression in Leydig cells inhibits steroidogenesis by down-regulating 3ß-hydroxysteroid dehydrogenase. J Endocrinol 185:507–517

Middendorff R, Davidoff MS, Holstein AF (1993) Neuroendocrine marker substances in human Leydig cells – changes by disturbances of testicular function. Andrologia 25:257–262

Middendorff R, Davidoff MS, Mayer B, Holstein AF (1995) Neuroendocrine characteristics of human Leydig cell tumors. Andrologia 27:351–355

Middendorff R, Müller D, Paust HJ, Davidoff MS, Mukhopadhyay AK (1996) Natriuretic peptides in the human testis: evidence for a potential role of C-type natriuretic peptide in Leydig cells. J Clin Endocrinol Metab 81:4324–4328

Middendorff R, Müller D, Paust HJ, Holstein AF, Davidoff MS (1997a) New aspects of Leydig cell function. Adv Exp Med Biol 424:125–138

Middendorff R, Müller D, Wichers S, Holstein AF, Davidoff MS (1997b) Evidence for production and functional activity of nitric oxide in seminiferous tubules and blood vessels of the human testis. J Clin Endocrinol Metab 82:4154–4161

Middendorff R, Müller D, Holstein AF (1997c) C-type natriuretic peptide (CNP) system in the testis: a physiological role of neuroactive factors in Leydig cells. Biomed Rev 8:111–117

Middendorff R, Davidoff MS, Behrends S, Mewe M, Miethens A, Müller D (2000a) Multiple roles of the messenger molecule cGMP in testicular function. Andrologia 32:55–59

Middendorff R, Kumm M, Davidoff MS, Holstein AF, Müller D (2000b) Generation of cyclic guanosine monophosphate by heme oxygenases in the human testis – a regulatory role for carbon monoxide in Sertoli cells? Biol Reprod 63:651–657

Middendorff R, Müller D, Mewe M, Mukhopadhyay AK, Holstein AF, Davidoff MS (2002) The tunica albuginea of the human testis is characterized by complex contraction and relaxation activities regulated by cyclic GMP. J Clin Endocrinol Metab 87:3486–3499

Mignone JL, Roig-Lopez JL, Fedtsova N, Schones DE, Manganas LN, Maletic-Savatic M, Keyes WM, Mills AA, Glieberman A, Zhang MQ, Enikolopov G (2007) Neural potential of a stem cell population in the hair follicle. Cell Cycle 6:2161–2170

Miñana MD, Carbonell-Uberos F, Mirabet V, Marin S, Encabo A (2008) IFATS collection: identification of hemangioblasts in the adult human adipose tissue. Stem Cells 26:2696–2704

Minasi MG, Riminucci M, De Angelis LC, Borello U, Berarducci B, Innocenzy A, Caprioli A, Sirabella D, Baiocchi M, De Maria R, Boratto R, Jaffredo T, Broccoli V, Bianco P, Cossu G (2002) The meso-angioblast: a multipotent, self-renewing cell that originates from the dorsal aorta differentiates into most mesodermal tissues. Development 129:2773–2783

Miura M, Gronthos S, Zhao M, Lu B, Fisher LW, Robey PG, Shi S (2003) SHED: stem cells from human exfoliated deciduous teeth. Proc Natl Acad Sci USA 100:5807–5812

Miura Y, Gao Z, Miura M, Seo B-M, Sonoyama W, Chen W, Gronthos S, Zhang L, Shi S (2006) Mesenchymal stem cells-organized bone marrow elements: an alternative hematopoietic progenitor resource. Stem Cells 24:2428–2436

Molenaar R, de Rooij DG, Rommerts FFG, Reuvers PJ, van der Molen HJ (1985) Specific destruction of Leydig cells in mature rats after in vivo administration of ethane dimethyl sulfonate. Biol Reprod 33:1213–1222

Molenaar R, Rommerts FF, van der Molen HJ (1986a) Non-specific esterase: a specific and useful marker enzyme for Leydig cells from mature rats. J Endocrinol 108:329–334

Molenaar R, de Rooij DG, Rommerts FF, van der Molen HJ (1986b) Repopulation of Leydig cells in mature rats after selective destruction of the existent Leydig cells with ethylene dimethane sulfonate is dependent on luteinizinig hormone and not follicle-stimulating hormone. Endocrinology 118:2546–2554

Mondillo C, Pagotto RM, Piotrkowski B, Reche CG, Patrignani ZJ, Cymeryng CB, Pignataro OP (2009) Involvement of nitric oxide synthase in the mechanism of histamine-induced inhibition of Leydig cell steroidogenesis via HRH1 receptor subtypes in Sprague-Dawley rats. Biol Reprod 80:144–152

Montagne J-J, Ladram A, Grouselle D, Nicolas P, Bulant M (1996) Identification and cellular localization of thyrotropin-releasing hormone-related peptides in rat testis. Endocrinology 137:185–191

Moore R, Laure L (2004) Cell surface molecules and truncal neural crest ontogeny: a perspective. Birth Defects Res Part C 72:140–150

Morikawa S, Baluk P, Kaidoh T, Haskell A, Jain RK, McDonals DM (2002) Abnormalities in pericytes on blood vessels and endothelial sprouts in tumors. Am J Pathol 160:985–1000

Morohashi K (1997) The ontogenesis of the steroidogenic tissues. Genes Cells 2:95–106

Morris AJ, Taylor MF, Morris ID (1997) Leydig cell apoptosis in response to ethane dimethanesulphonate after both in vivo and in vitro treatment. J Androl 18:274–280

Morris ID, Phillips DM, Bardin CW (1986) Ethylene dimethanesulfonate destroys Leydig cells in the rat testis. Endocrinology 118:709–719

Morrison SJ, Spreadling AC (2008) Stem cells and niches: mechanisms that promote stem cell maintenance throughot live. Cell 132:598–611

Morrison SJ, White PM, Zock C, Anderson DJ (1999) Prospective identification, isolation by flow cytometry, and in vivo self-renewal of multipotent mammalian neural stem cells. Cell 96:37–749

Morrow EM, Furukawa T, Lee JE, Cepko CL (1999) NeuroD regulates multiple functions in the developing neural retina in rodent. Development 126:23–36

Muffler S, Stark HJ, Falkowska-Hansen B, Bohenke K, Bühring HJ, Marmé A, Bickenbach JR, Boukamp P (2008) A stable niche supports long-term maintenance of human epidermal stem cells in organotypic cultures. Stem Cells 26:2506–2515

Mujtaba T, Mayer-Proschel M, Rao MS (1998) A common neural progenitor for CNS and PNS. Dev Biol 200:1–15

Mukhopadhyay AK, Bohnet HG, Leidenberger FA (1986) Testosterone production by mouse Leydig cells is stimulated in vitro by atrial natriuretic factor. FEBS Lett 202:111–116

Mukhopadhyay AK, Cobilanschi J, Brunswig-Spickenheier B, Leidenberger FA (1995) Relevance of the tissue prorenin-renin-angiotensin system to male reproductive physiology. In: Mukhopadhyay AK, Raizada MK (eds) Tissue renin-angiotensin systems. current concepts of local regulators in reproductive and endocrine organs. Plenum, New York, pp 269–277

Müller D, Middendorff R, Davidoff MS (1999) Neurotrophic factors in the testis. Biomed Rev 10:25–30

Müller D, Cortes-Dericks L, Budnik LT, Brunswig-Spickenheier B, Pancratius M, Speth RC, Mukhopadhyay AK, Middendorff R (2006a) Homologous and lysophosphatidic acid-induced desensitization of the atrial natriuretic peptide receptor, guanylyl cyclase-A, in MA-10 Leydig cells. Endocrinology 147:2974–2985

Müller D, Davidoff MS, Bargheer O, Paust H-J, Pusch W, Koeva Y, Ježek D, Holstein AF, Middendorff R (2006b) The expression of neurotrophins and their receptors in the prenatal and adult human testis: evidence for functions in Leydig cells. Histochem Cell Biol 126:199–211

Müller SM, Stolt CC, Terzowski G, Blum C, Amagai T, Kessaris N, Iannarelli P, Richardson WD, Wegner M, Rodewald H-R (2008) Neural crest origin of perivascular mesenchyme in the adult thymus. J Immunol 180:5344–5351

Murray TJ, Fowler PA, Abramovich DR, Haites N, Lea RG (2000) Human fetal testis: second trimester proliferative and steroidogenic capacities. J Clin Endocrinol Metab 85:4812–4817

Murakami T, Uno Y, Ohtsuka A, Taguchi T (1989) The blood vascular architecture of the rat testis: a scanning electron microscopic study of corrosion casts followed by light microscopy of tissue sections. Arch Histol Cytol 52:151–172

Murono EP, Washburn AL, Goforth DP, Wu N (1992) Evidence for basic fibroblast growth factor receptors in cultured immature Leydig cells. Mol Cell Endocrinol 88:39–45

Myers RB, Abney TO (1991) Interstitial cell proliferation in the testis of the ethylene dimethane sulfonate-treated rat. Steroids 56:91–96

Nadin BM, Goodell MA, Hirshi KK (2003) Phenotype and hematopoietic potential of side population cells throughout embryonic development. Blood 102:2436–2443

Nagano T, Suzuki F (1976) Freeze-fracture observations on the intercellular junctions of Sertoli cells and of Leydig cells in the human testis. Cell Tissue Res 166:37–48

Nardi NB (2005) All the adult stem cells, where do they all come from? An external source for organ-specific stem cell pools. Med Hypotheses 64:811–817

Nayernia K, Lee JH, Drusenheimer N, Nolte J, Wulf G, Dressel R, Gromoll J, Engel W (2006) Derivation of male germ cells from bone marrow stem cells. Lab Invest 86:654–663

Neaves WB (1975) Leydig cells. A Report Prepated for The Ford Foundation Review of Research and Support in Reproductive Biology and Contrarceptive Development. Contraceptive 11:571–606

Nee Pathak ND, Lal B (2008) Nitric oxide: an autocrine regulator of Leydig cell steroidogenesis in the Asian catfish, Clarias betrachus. Gen Comp Endocrinol 158:161–167

Nef S, Schaad O, Stallings NR, Cederooth CR, Pitetti J-L, Schaer G, Malki S, Dubois-Dauphin M, Boizet-Bonhourse B, Descombes P, Parker KL, Vassalli J-D (2005) Gene expression during sex determination reveals a robust genetic program at the onset of ovarian development. Dev Biol 287:361–377

Ng TB, Ooi VEC (1990) Effect of pineal indoles on testicular histology in mice. Arch Androl 25:137–145

Nehls V, Drenckhahn D (1993) The versatility of microvascular pericytes: from mesenchyme to smooth muscle? Histochemistry 99:1–12

Nes WD, Lukyanenko Y, Jia ZH, Quideau S, Howald WN, Pratum TK, West RR, Hutson JC (2000) Identification of the lipophilic factor produced by macrophages that stimulates steroidogenesis. Endocrinology 141:953–958

Neumann A, Haider SG, Hilscher B (1993) Temporal coincidence of the appearance of elongated spermatids and histochemical reaction of 11ß-hydroxysteroid dehydrogenase in rat Leydig cells. Andrologia 25:263–269

Niki T, Pekny M, Hellemans K, Bleser PD, Berg KV, Vaeyens F, Quartier E, Schuit F, Geers A (1999) Class VI intermediate filament protein nestin is induced during activation of rat hepatic stellate cells. Hepathology 29:520–527

Nikolova G, Lammert E (2003) Interdependent development of blood vessels and organs. Cell Tissue Res 314:33–42

Nikolova G, Jabs N, Konstantinova I, Domogatskaya A, Tryggvason K, Sorokin L, Fässler R, Gu G, Gerber H-P, Ferrara N, Melton DA, Lammert E (2006a) The vascular basement membrane: a niche for insulin gene expression and ß-cell proliferation. Dev Cell 10:397–405

Nikolova G, Strilic B, Lammert E (2006b) The vascular niche and its basement membrane. Trends Cell Biol 17:19–25

Nishikawa SI, Osawa M (2006) What is a stem cell niche. Ernst Schering Res Found Workshop 60:1–14

Nishimura R, Kondo I (1964) Morphological study of the interstitial tissue of the testicles. Urol Int 18:1–24

Nishino K, Yamanouchi K, Naito K, Tojo H (2001) Characterization of mesonephric cells that migrate into the XY gonad during differentiation. Exp Cell Res 267:225–232

Nobuhisa I, Ohtsu N, Okada S, Nakagata N, Taga T (2007) Identification of a population of cells with hematopoietic stem cell properties in mouse aorta-gonad-mesonephros cultures. Exp Cell Res 313:965–974

Nussbaum M (1880) Zur Differenzierung des Geschlechts im Tierreich. Arch Mikrosk Anat 18:1–121

O'Donnell L, Robertson KM, Jones ME, Simpson ER (2001) Estrogen and spermatogenesis. Endocr Rev 22:289–318

Oh H, Bradfute SB, Gallardo TD, Nakamura T, Gaussin V, Mishina Y, Pocius J, Michael LH, Behringer RR, Garry DJ, Entman ML (2003) Cardiac progenitor cells from adult myocardium: homing, differentiation, and fusion after infarction. Proc Natl Acad Sci USA 100:12313–12318

Ohneda O, Fennie C, Zheng Z, Donahue C, La H, Villacorta R, Cairns B, Lasky LA (1998) Hematopoietic stem cell maintenance and differentiation are supported by embryonic aorta-gonad-mesonephros region-derived endothelium. Blood 92:908–919

Ohyama M (2007) Hair follicle bulge: a fascinating reservoir of epithelial stem cells. J Dermatol Sci 46:81–89

Oishi K, Ogawa Y, Gamoh S, Uchida MK (2002) Contractile responses of smooth muscle cells differentiated from rat neural stem cells. J Physiol 540:139–152

Okano H (2002a) Stem cell biology of the central nervous system. J Neurosci Res 69:698–707

Okano H (2002b) Neural stem cells: progression of basic research and perspective for clinical application. Kejo J Med 51:115–128

Olivares AN, Valladares LE, Bustos-Obregon E, Nunez SM (1989) Testicular function of sexually immature rats chronically treated with melatonin. Arch Biol Med Exp 22:387–393

Olson L, Ayer-LeLievre C, Ebendal T, Seiger A (1987) Nerve growth factor-like immunoreactivities in rodent salivary glands and testis. Cell Tissue Res 248:275–286

Oostendorp RA, Narvey KN, Kusadasi N, de Bruijn MFTR, Saris C, Ploemacher RE, Medvinsky AL, Dzierzak EA (2002) Stromal cell lines from mouse aorta-gonad-mesonephros subregions are potent supporters of hematopoietic stem cell activity. Blood 99:1183–1189

Ortiz-Gonzalez XR, Keene CD, Verfaillie CM, Low WC (2004) Neural induction of adult bone marrow and umbilical cord stem cells. Curr Neurovasc Res 1:207–213

O'Shaughnessy PJ, Willerton L, Bakcr PJ (2002) Changes in Leydig cell gene expression during development in the mouse. Biol Reprod 66:966–975

O'Shaughnessy PJ, Baker PJ, Johnston H (2006) The foetal Leydig cell – differentiation, function and regulation. Int J Androl 29:90–95

O'Shaughnessy PJ, Baker PJ, Monteiro A, Cassie S, Bhattacharya S, Fowler PA (2007a) Developmental changes in human fetal testicular cell numbers and messenger ribonucleic acid levels during the second trimester. J Clin Endocrinol Metab 92:4792–4801

O'Shaughnessy PJ, Johnston H, Baker PJ (2007b) Development of Leydig cell steroidogenesis. In: Payne AH, Hardy MP (eds) Contemporarry endocrinology: the Leydig cell in health and disease. Humana, Totowa, 173–179

O'Shaughnessy PJ, Hu L, Baker PJ (2008a) Effect of germ cell depletion on levels of specific mRNA transcripts in mouse Sertoli cells and Leydig cells. Reproduction 135:839–850

O'Shaughnessy PJ, Morris ID, Baker PJ (2008b) Leydig cell re-generation and expression of cell signalling molecules in the germ cell-free testis. Reproduction 135:851–858

Ozerdem U, Stallcup WB (2003) Early contribution of pericytes to angiogenic sprouting and tube formation. Angiogenesis 6:241–249

Ozerdem U, Grako KA, Dahlin-Huppe K, Monosov E, Stallcup WB (2001) NG2 proteoglycan is expressed exclusively by mural cells during vascular morphogenesis. Dev Dyn 222:218–227

Pablos JL, Amara A, Bouloc A, Santjago B, Caruz A, Galindo M, Delaunay T, Virelizier L, Arenzana-Seisdedos F (1999) Stromal-cell derived factor is expressed by dendritic cells and endothelium in human skin. Am J Pathol 155:1577–1586

Packer MA, Stasiv Y, Benraiss A, Chmielinicki E, Grinberg A, Westphal H, Goldman SA, Enikolopov G (2003) Nitric oxide negatively regulates mammalian adult neurogenesis. Proc Natl Acad Sci USA 100:9566–9571

Palmer TD, Willhoite AR, Gage FH (2000) Vascular niche for adult hippocampal neurogenesis. J Comp Neurol 425:479–494

Pandey KH, Orgebin-Crist MC (1991) Atrial natriuretic factor in mammalian testis: immunological detection in spermatozoa. Biochem Biophys Res Commun 180:437–444

Pandey KN, Misono KS, Inagami T (1984) Evidence for intracellular formation of angiotensins: coexistence of renin and angiotensin-converting enzyme in Leydig cells. Biochem Biophys Res Commun 122:1337–1343

Pandey KN (1994) Atrial natriuretic factor inhibits the phosphorylation of protein kinase C in plasma membrane preparations of cultured Leydig tumor cells. J Androl 15:100–109

Paniagua R, Rodriguez MC, Nistal M, Fraile B, Regadera J, Amat P (1988) Changes in surface area and number of Leydig cells in relation to the 6 stages of the cycle of the human seminiferous epithelium. Anat Embryol 178:423–427

Park C-S, Park R, Krishna G (1996) Constitutive expression and structural diversity of inducible isoform of nitric oxide synthase in human tissues. Life Set 59:219–225

Park I-H, Zhao R, West JA, Yabbuchi A, Huo H, Ince TA, Lerou PH, Lensch MW, Daley GQ (2008) Reprogramming of human somatic cells to pluripotency with defined factors. Nature 451:141–147

Park SY, Jameson JL (2005) Transcriptional regulation of gonadal development and differentiation. Endocrinology 146:1035–1042

Park SY, Tong M, Jameson JL (2007) Distinct roles for steroidogenic factor 1 and desert hedgehog pathways in fetal and adult Leydig cell development. Endicrinology 148:3704–3710

Parvinen M (1982) Regulation of the seminiferous epithelium. Endocr Rev 6:663–671

Passino MA, Adams RA, Sikorski SL, Akassoglou K (2007) Regulation of hepatic stellate cell differentiation by the neurotrophin receptor p75NTR. Science 315:1853–1856

Paus R, Ark P, Tiede S (2008) (Neuro-)endocrinology of epithelial hair follicle cells. Mol Cell Endocrinol 288:38–51

Payne AH (2007) Steroidogenic enzymes in Leydig cells. In: Payne AH, Hardy MP (eds) Contemporarry endocrinology: the Leydig cell in health and disease. Humana, Totowa, 157–171

Payne AH, O'Shaughnessy PJ (1996) Structure, function and regulation of steroidogenic enzymes In: Payne AH, Hardy MP, Russel LD (eds) The Leydig cell. Cache River, Vienna, pp 259–285

Pearse AGE (1969) The cytochemistry and ultrastructure of polypeptide hormone-producing cells of the APUD series and the embryonic, physiologic and pathologic implications of the concept. J Histochem Cytochem 17:303–313

Pearse AGE (1986) The diffuse neuroendocrine system: peptides, amines, placodes and the APUD theory. Prog Brain Res 68:25–31

Péault B, Rudnicki M, Torrente Y, Cossu G, Tremblay JP, Partridge T, Gussoni E, Kunkel LM, Huard J (2007) Stem and progenitor cells in skeletal muscle development, maintenance, and therapy. Mol Ther 15:867–877

Pelletier G, Li S, Luu-The V, Tremblay Y, Bélanger A, Labrie F (2001) Immunoelectron microscopic localization of three key steroidogenic enzymes (cytochrome P450scc, 3ß-hydroxysteroid dehydrogenase and cytochrome P450c17) in rat adrenal cortex and gonads. J Endocrinol 171:373–383

Pelliniemi LJ, Kuopio T, Fröjdman K (1996) The cell biology and function of the fetal Leydig cells. In: Payne AH, Hardy MP, Russell LD (eds) The Leydig cell. Cache River Press, Vienna, IL, pp 143–158

Peng H, Huard J (2004) Muscle-derived stem cells for musculoskeletal tissue regeneration and repair. Transplant Immunol 12:311–319

Pereira VM, Costa AP, Rosa-E-Silva AA, Vieira MA, Reis AM (2008) Regulation of steroidogenesis by atrial natriuretic peptide (ANP) in the rat testis: differential involvement of GC-A and C receptors. Peptides 29:2024–2032

Perez-Armendariz EM, Romano MC, Luna J, Miranda C, Bennett MVL, Moreno AP (1994) Characterization of gap junctions between pairs of Leydig cells from mouse testis. Am J Physiol 267:C570–C580

Peters HK (1977) Die Ultrastruktur heterotoper Leydigzellen beim Menschen. Andrologia 9:337–348

Petersen BE, Bowen WC, Patrene KD, Mars WM, Sullivan AK, Murase N, Boggs SS, Greenberger JS, Goff JP (1999) Bone marrow as a potential source of hepatic oval cells. Science 284:1168–1170

Petersen BE, Groosbard B, Hatch H, Pi L, Deng J, Scott EW (2003) Mouse A6-positive hepatic oval cells also express several hematopoietic stem cell markers. Hepatology 37:632–640

Petkova-Kirova P, Rakovska A, Della Corte L, Radomirov R, Mayer A (2008) Neurotensin modulation of acetylcholine, GABA, and aspartate release from rat prefrontal cortex studied in vivo with microdialysis. Brain Res Bull 77:129–135

Peunova N, Enikolopov G (1995) Nitric oxide triggers a switch to growth arrest during differentiation of neuronal cells. Nature 375:68–73

Pierret C, Spears K, Maruniak JA, Kirk MD (2006) Neural crest as the source of adult stem cells. Stem Cells Dev 15:286–291

Pla P, Larue L (2003) Involvement of endothelin receptors in normal and pathological development of neural crest cells. Int J Dev Biol 47:315–325

Pla P, Moore R, Morali OG, Grille S, Martinozzi S, Delmas V, Larue L (2001) Cadherins in neural cell development and transformation. J Cell Physiol 189:121–132

Plato J (1896) Die interstitiellen Zellen des Hodens und ihrer physiologische Bedeutung. Arch Mikrosk Anat 48:280–304

Plato J (1897) Zur Kenntnis der Anatomie und Physiologie der Geschlechtsorgane. Arch Mikrosk Anat 50:640–685

Pinzani M, Failli P, Ruocco C, Casini A, Milani S, Baldi E, Giotti A, Gentillni P (1992) Fat-storing cells as liver-specific pericytes. Spatial dynamics of agonist-stimulated calcium transients. J Clin Invest 90:642–646

Pouget C, Gautier R, Teillet M-A, Jaffredo T (2006) Somite-derived cell replace ventral aortic hemangioblasts and provide aortic smooth muscle cells of the trunk. Development 133:1013–1022

Pouget C, Pottin K, Jaffredo T (2008) Sclerotomal origin of vascular smooth muscle cells and pericytes in the embryo. Dev Biol 315:437–447

Prince FP (2001) The triphasic nature of Leydig cell development in humans, and comments on nomenclature. J Endocrinol 168:213–216

Prince FP (2007) The human Leydig cell. Functional morphology and developmental history. In: Payne AH, Hardy MP (eds) Contemporarry endocrinology: the Leydig cell in health and disease. Humana, Totowa, pp 71–89

Pudney J (1996) Comparative cytology of the Leydig cell. In: Payne AH, Hardy MP, Russell LD (eds) The Leydig cell. Cache River, Vienna, pp 97–142

Puglianiello A, Campagnolo L, Farini D, Cipollone D, Russo MA, Siracusa G (2004) Expression and role of PDGF-BB and PDGF-ß during testis morphogenesis in the mouse embryo. J Cell Sci 117:1151–1160

Purvis K, Clausen OPF, Ulvil NM, Hansson V (1979) Functional and morphological characteristics of rat Leydig cells: effects of prepubertal and postpubertal structure and function. In: Sternberger A, Sternberger E (eds) Testicular development. Raven, New York, pp 212–215

Qian Y-M, Song W-C (1999) Regulation of estrogen sulfotransferase expression in Leydig cells by cyclic adenosine 3′,5′-monophosphate and androgen. Endocrinology 140:1048–1053

Qu-Petersen Z, Deasy B, Jankowski R, Ikezawa M, Cummins J, Pruchnic R, Mytinger J, Cao B, Gates C, Wernig A, Huard J (2002) Identification of a novel population of muscle stem cells in mice: potential for muscle regeneration. J Cell Biol 157:851–864

Raburn DJ, Coquelin A, Hutson JC (1991) Human chorionic gonadotropin increases the concentration of macrophages in neonatal rat testis. Biol Reprod 45:172–177

Raeside JI, Christie HL, Renaud TL, Sinclair PA (2006) The boar testis: the most versatile steroid producing organ known. Soc Reprod Fertil Suppl 62:85–97

Rajan P, Panchision DM, Newell LF, McKay RDG (2003) BMPs signal alternately through a SMAD or FRAP-STAT pathway to regulate fate choice in CNS stem cells. J Cell Biol 161:911–921

Rajantie I, Ilmonen M, Alminaite A, Ozerdem U, Alitalo K, Salven P (2004) Adult bone marrow-derived cells recruited during angiogenesis comprise precursors for periendothelial vascular mural cells. Blood 104:2084–2086

Ramalho-Santos M, Yoon S, Matsuzaki Y, Milligan RC, Melton DA (2002) "Stemness": transcriptional profiling of embryonic and adult stem cells. Science 298:597–600

Rao JN, Debeljuk L, Bartke A (1995) Effects of tachykinins on the secretory activity of rat Sertoli cells in vitro. Endocrinology 136:1315–1318

Rao M (2004a) Stem and precursor cells in the nervous system. J Neurotrauma 21:415–427

Rao M (2004b) Stem sense: a proposal for the classification of stem cells. Stem Cells Dev 13:452–455

Rasmusen AT (1932) Interstitial cells of the testis. In: Cowdrey EV (ed) Special cytology vol 3. Hafner, New York, pp 1675–1725

Ratajczak MZ, Zuba-Surma EK, Wysoczynski M, Ratajczak J, Kucia M (2008) Very small embryonic-like stem cells: characterization, developmental origin, and biological significance. Exp Hematol 36:742–751

Real C, Glavieux-Pardanaud C, Vaigot P, Le Douarin NM, Dupin E (2005) The Instability of the neural crest phenotypes: Schwann cells can differentiate into myofibroblasts. Int J Dev Biol 49:151–159

Real C, Glavieux-Pardanaud C, Le Douarin NM, Dupin E (2006) Clonally cultured differentiated pigmented cells can differentiate and generate multipotent progenitors with self-renewing potential. Dev Biol 300:656–669

Regadera J, Kobo P, Martinez-Garzia F, Nistal M, Paniagua R (1993) Testosterone immunoexpression in human Leydig cells of the tunica albuginea testis and spermatic cord. A quantitative study in normal foetuses, young adults, elderly men and patients with cryptorchidism. Andrologia 25:115–122

Regaud C, Policard A (1901) Etude comparative du testicule du porc normal, impubère et ectopique, au point de vue des cellules interstitielles. C R Soc Biol 53:450–452

Reinke F (1896) Beiträge zur Histologie des Menschen. Arch Mikrosk Anat 47:34–44

Remy-Martin JP, Marandin A, Challier B, Bernard G, Deschaseaux M, Herve P, Wei Y, Tsuji T, Auerbach R, Dennis JE, Moore KA, Greenberger JS, Charbord P (1999) Vascular smooth muscle differentiation of murine stroma: a sequential model. Exp Hematol 27:1782–1795

Reyes M, Lund T, Lencik T, Agular D, Koodie L, Verfaillie CM (2001) Purification and ex vivo expansion of postnatal human marrow mesodermal progenitor cells. Blood 98:2615–2625

Reyes M, Dudek A, Jahagirdar B, Koodie L, Marker PH, Verfaillie CM (2002) Origin of endothelial progenitors in human postnatal bone marrow. J Clin Invest 109:337–343

Reyes A, Moran CA, Suster S, Michal M, Dominquez H (2003) Neuroendocrine carcinomas (carcinoid tumors) of the testis. A clinicopathologic and immunohistochemical study of ten cases. Am J Clin Pathol 120:182–187

Rietze RL, Valcanis H, Brooker GF, Thomas T, Voss AK, Bartlett PF (2001) Purification of a pluripotent neural stem cell from the adult mouse brain. Nature 412 (6848):736–739

Risbridger GP (1996) Regulation of Leydig cells by inhibins and activins. In: Payne AH, Hardy MP, Russell LD (eds) The Leydig cell. Cache River, Vienna, pp 493–506

Roberts GW, Allen YS (1986) Immunohistochemistry of brain neuropeptides. In: Polak JM, Van Noorden S (eds) Immunocytochemistry. Modern methods and applications. Wright, Bristol, pp 339–350

Rochefort GY, Delorme G, Lopez A, Hérault O, Bonnet P, Charbord P, Eder V, Domenech J (2006) Multipotential mesenchymal stem cells are mobilized into peripheral blood by hypoxia. Stem Cells 24:2202–2208

Romeo R, Pelliteri R, Russo A, Marcello MF (2004) Catecholaminergic phenotype of human Leydig cells. Ital J Anat Embryol 109:45–54

Roosen-Runge EC, Anderson D (1959) The development of the interstitial cells in the testis of the albino rat. Acta Anat 37:125–137

Rosenthal N (2003) Prometeus's vulture and the stem-cell promise. N Engl J Med 349:267–274

Roskams T, Cassiman D, De Vos R, Libbrecht L (2004) Neuroregulation of neuroendocrine compartment of the liver. Anat Rec A 280A:910–923

Ross AJ, Capel B (2005) Signaling at the crossroads of gonad development. Trends Endocrinol Metab 16:19–25

Rosselli M, Keller PJ, Dubey RK (1998) Role of nitric oxide in the biology, physiology and pathophysiology of reproduction. Hum Reprod Update 4:3–24

Rouleau MF, Mitchell J, Goltzman D (1990) Characterization of the major parathyroid hormone target cell in the endosteal metaphysic of rat long bones. J Bone Miner Res 5:1043–1053

Rucker HK, Wynder HJ, Thomas WE (2000) Cellular mechanisms of CNS pericytes. Brain Res Bull 51:363–369

Ruffoli R, Giambelluca MA, Giannessi F, Soldani P, Grasso L, Gasperi M, Giannessi F (2001) Ultrastructural localization of the NADPH-diaphorase activity in the Leydig cells of aging mice. Anat Embryol 203:383–391

Russell LD (1996) Mammalian Leydig cell structure. In: Payne AH, Hardy MP, Russell LD (eds) The Leydig cell. Cache River, Vienna, pp 43–96

Russell LD, Amlani SR, Vogel AW, Weber JE (1981) Characterization of filaments within Leydig cells of the rat testis. Am J Anat 178:231–240

Russell LD, de Franca LR, Hess R, Cooke P (1995) Characteristics of mitotic cells in developing and adult testes with observations on cell lineages. Tissue Cell 27:105–128

Russo MA, Odorisio T, Fradeani A, Rienzi L, De Felici M, Cattanaeo A, Siracusa G (1994) Low-affinity nerve growth factor receptor is expressed during testicular morphogenesis and in germ cells at specific stages of spermatogenesis. Mol Reprod Dev 37:157–166

Sabatini F, Petecchia L, Tavian M, Jodon de Villeroché V, Rossi GA, Brouty-Boyé D (2005) Human bronchial fibroblasts exhibit a mesenchymal stem cell phenotype and multilienage differentiating potentialities. Lab Invest 85:962–971

Sadovsky Y, Crawford PA, Woodson KG, Polish JA, Clements MA, Tourtellotte LM, Simburger K, Milbrandt J (1995) Mice deficient in the orphan receptor steroidogenic factor 1 lack adrenal gland and gonads but express P450 side-chain-cleavage enzyme in the placenta and have normal embryonic serum levels of corticosteroids. Proc Natl Acad Sci USA 92:10939–10943

Saez JM (1994) Leydig cells: endocrine, paracrine, and autocrine regulation. Endocr Rev 15:574–626

Saez JM, Lejeune H (1996) Regulation of Leydig cell functions by hormones and growth factors other than LH and IGF-1. In: Payne AH, Hardy MP, Russell LD (eds) The Leydig cell. Cache River, Vienna, pp 383–406

Saez JM, Lejeune H, Avallet O, Habert R, Durand P (1995) Le contrôle des functions différenciés des cellules de Leydig. Med Sci 11:547–553

Sahlgren CM, Mikhailov A, Hellman J, Chou Y-H, Lendahl U, Goldman RD, Ericsson JE (2001) Mitotic reorganization of the intermediate filament protein nestin involves phosphorylation by cdc2 kinase. J Biol Chem 276:16456–16463

Sainson RCA, Harris AL (2008) Regulation of angiogenesis by homotypic and heterotypic notch signalling in endothelial cells and pericytes: from basic research to potential therapies. Angiogenesis 11:41–51

Saint-Pol P, Peyrat JP, Engelhardt RP, Leroy-Martin B (1986) Immunohistochemical localization of enkephalins in adult rat testis: evidence for a gonadotropin control. Andrologia 18:485–488

Sampoalesi M, Torrente Y, Innocenzi A, Tonlorenzi R, D'Antona G, Pellegrino MA, Barresi R, Bresolin N, De Angelis MGC, Campbell KP, Bottinelli R, Cossu G (2003) Cell therapy of α-sarcoglycan null dystrophic mice through intra-arterial delivery of mesangioblasts. Science 301:487–492

Sarugaser R, Lickorish D, Baksh D, Hosseini MM, Davies JE (2005) Human umbilical cord perivascular (HUCPV) cells: a source of mesenchymal progenitors. Stem Cells 23:220–229

Sato M, Suzuki S, Senoo H (2003) Hepatic stellate cells: unique characterisrics in cell biology and phenotype. Cell Struct Funct 28:105–112

Sato S, Braham CS, Putnam SK, Hull EM (2005) Neuronal nitric oxide synthase and gonadal steroid interaction in the MPOA of male rats: co-localization and testosterone-induced restoration of copulation and nNOS-immunoreactivity. Brain Res 1043:205–213

Saxena R, Theise N (2004) Canalis of Hering: recent insights and current knowledge. Semin Liver Dis 24:43–48

Scehnet JF, Jiang W, Kumar SR, Krasnoperov V, Trindade A, Benedito R, Djokovic D, Borges C, Ley EJ, Duarte A, Gill PS (2007) Inhibition of Dll4-mediated signalling induces proliferation of immature vessels and results in poor tissue perfusion. Blood 109:4753–4760

Schäfers BA, Schlutius BG, Haider SG (2001) Ontogenesis of oxidadtive reaction of 17ß-hydroxysteroid dehydrogenase and 11ß-hydroxysteroid dehydrogenase in rat Leydig cells, a histochemical study. Histochem J 33:585–595

Schmahl J, Eicher EM, Washburn LL, Capel B (2000) Sry induces cell proliferation in the mouse gonad. Development 127:65–73

Schneider S, Bosse F, D'Urso D, Muller H, Sereda MW, Nave K, Niehaus A, Kemp T, Schnolzer M, Trotter J (2001) The AG2 protein is a novel marker for the Schwann cell lineage expressed by immature and nonmyelinating Schwann cells. J Neurosci 21:920–933

Schulze C (1984) Sertoli cells and Leydig cells in man. Adv Anat Embryol Cell Biol 88:1–104

Schulze C, Holstein AF (1978) Leydig cells within the lamina propria of seminiferous tubules in four patients with azoospermia. Andrologia 10:444–452

Schulze W, Davidoff MS, Holstein AF (1987a) Are Leydig cells of neural origin? Substance P-like immunoreactivity in human testicular tissue. Acta Endocrinol 115:373–377

Schulze W, Davidoff MS, Holstein AF, Schirren C (1987b) Processing of testicular biopsies fixed in Stieve's solution for visualization of substance P- and methionine-enkephalin-immunoreactifvity in Leydig cells. Andrologia 19:419–422

Schulze W, Davidoff MS, Ivell R, Holstein AF (1991) Neuron specific enolase-like immunoreactivity in human Leydig cells. Andrologia 23:279–283

Schumacher H, Müller D, Mukhopadhyay AK (1992) Stimulation of testosterone production by atrial natriuretic peptide in isolated mouse Leydig cells results from a promiscuous activation of cyclic AMP-dependent protein kinase by cyclic GMP. Mol Cell Endocrinol 90:47–52

Schumacher H, Matsuda Y, Mukhopadhyay AK (1993) HS-142-1 inhibits testosterone production and guanosine-3',5'-cyclic monophosphate accumulation stimulated by atrial natriuretic peptide in isolated mouse Leydig cells. Mol Cell Endocrinol 94:105–110

Schwartz RE, Reyes M, Koodie, Jiang Y, Blackstad M, Lund T, Lenvik T, Johnson S, Hu W-S, Verfaillie CM (2002) Multipotent adult progenitor cells from the bone marrow differentiate into functional hepatocyte-like cells. J Clin Invest 109:1291–1302

Seidl K, Buchberger A, Erck A (1996) Expression of nerve growth factor and neurotrophin receptors in testicular cells suggest novel roles for neurotrophins outside the nervous system. Reprod Fertil Dev 8:1075–1087

Sejersen T, Lendahl U (1993) Transient expression of the intermediate filament nestin during skeletal muscle development. J Cell Sci 106:1291–1300

Sekido R, Lovell-Badge R (2008) Sex determination involves synergistic action of SRY and SF1 on a specific Sox9 enhancer. Nature 453:930–934

Shaha C, Liotta AS, Krieger DT, Bardin CW (1984) The ontogeny of immunoreactive beta-endorphin in fetal, neonatal, and pubertal testes from mouse and hamster. Endocrinology 114:1584–1591

Shan L-X, Hardy MP (1992) Developmental changes in levels of luteinizing hormone receptor and androgen receptor in rat Leydig cells. Endocrinology 131:1107–1114

Shan L-X, Hardy DO, Catterall JF, Hardy MP (1995a) Effects of luteinizing hormone (LH) and androgen on steady state levels of messenger ribonucleic acid for LH receptors, androgen receptors, and steroidogenic enzymes in rat Leydig cell progenitors in vivo. Endocrinology 136:1686–1693

Shan L-X, Bardin CW, Hardy MP (1997) Immunohistochemical analysis of androgen effects on androgen receptor expression in developing Leydig and Sertoli cells. Endocrinology 138:1259–1266

Sharpe RM (1983) Local control of testicular function. Q J Exp Physiol 68:265–287

Sharpe RM (1986) Paracrine control of the testis. Clin Endocr Metabl 15:185–207

Sharpe RM (1990) Intratesticular control of spermatogenesis. Clin Endocrinol 33:787–807

Sharpe RM (1993) Experimental evidence for Sertoli-germ cell and Sertoli-Leydig cell interactions. In: Russel LD, Grieswold MD (eds) The Sertoli cell. Cache River, Clearwater, pp 391–418

Sharpe RM (1994) Regulation of spermatogenesis. In: E Knobil, JD Neil (eds) The physiology of reproduction, 2nd edn. Raven, New York, pp 1363–1434

Sharpe RM, Cooper I (1987) Comparison of the effects on purified Leydig cells of four hormones (oxytocin, vasopressin, opioids and LHRH) with suggested paracrine roles in the testis. J Endocrinol 113:89–96

Sharpe RM, Rivas A, Walker M, McKinnell C, Fisher JS (2003) Effect of neonatal treatment of rats with potent or weak (environmental) oestrogens, or with a GnRH antagonist, on Leydig cell development and function through puberty into adulthood. Int J Androl 26:26–36

Shi S, Gronthos S (2003) Perivascular niche of postnatal mesenchymal stem cells in human bone marrow and dental pulp. J Bone Miner Res 18:696–704

Shih C-C, Weng Y, Mamelak A, LeBon T, Hu M.C.-T, Forman SJ (2001) Identification of a candidate human neurohematopoiedtic stem-cell population. Blood 98:2412–2422

Shihabuddin LS, Horner PJ, Ray J, Gage FH (2000) Adult spinal cord stem cells generate neurons after transplantation in the adult dentate gyrus. J Neurosci 20:8727–8735

Shimizu Y, Motohashi N, Iseki H, Kunita S, Sugiyama F, Ygami K-I (2006) A novel subpopulation lacking Oct4 expression in the testicular side population. Int J Mol Med 17:21–28

Shovlin TC, Durcova-Hills G, Surani A, McLaren A (2008) Heterogeneity in imprinted methylation patterns of pluripotent embryonic germ cells derived from pre-migratory mouse germ cells. Dev Biol 313:674–681

Shu W, Jiang YQ, Lu MM, Morrisey EE (2002) Wnt7b regulates mesenchymal proliferation and vascular development in the lung. Development 129:4831–4842

Sieber-Blum M, Grim M (2004a) The adult hair follicle: cradle for pluripotent neural crest stem cells. Birth Defects Res Part C 72:162–172

Sieber-Blum M, Hu Y (2008) Epidermal neural crest stem cells (EPI-NCSC) and pluripotency. Stem Cell Rev 4:256–260

Sieber-Blum M, Grim M, Hu YF, Szeder V (2004b) Pluripotent neural crest stem cells in the adult hair follicle. Dev Dyn 231:258–269

Sjöberg G, Jiang W-Q, Ringertz NR, Lendahl U, Sejersen T (1994) Colocalization of nestin and vimentin in skeletal muscle cells demonstrated by three-dimensional fluorescence digital imaging microscopy. Exp Cell Res 214:447–458

Sims DE (1986) The pericyte – a review. Tissue Cell 18:153–174

Sims DE (1991) Recent advances in pericyte biology – implications for health and disease. Can J Cardiol 7:431–443

Skinner MK, Fritz IB (1986) Identification of a non-mitogenic paracrine factor involved in mesenchymal-epithelial cell interaction between testicular peritubular cells and Sertoli cells. Mol Cell Endocrinol 44:85–97

Sklebar D, Semanjski K, Kos M, Sklebar I, Jezek D (2008) Foetal Leydig cells and the neuroendocrine system. Coll Antropol 32(Suppl 1):149–153

Slack JMW (2000) Stem cells in epithelial tissues. Science 287:1431–1433

Slusher BS, Zacco AE, Maslanski JA, Norris TE, McLane MW, Moore WG, Rogers NE, Ignarro LJ (1994) The cloned neurotensin receptor mediates cyclic GMP formation when coexpressed with nitric oxide synthase cDNA. Mol Pharmacol 46:115–121

Smet PJ, Edyvane KA, Jonavicius J, Marshall VR (1994) Colocalization of nitric oxide synthase with vasoactive intestinal peptide, neuropeptide Y, and thyrosine hydroxylase in nerves supplying the human ureter. Urol 152:1292–1296

Sobhan-Sarbandi D, Holstein AF (1988) Derivatives of the neural crest in the human spermatic cord. In: Holstein AF, Leidenberger F, Hölzer KH, Bettendorf G (eds) Carl Schirren symposium: advances in andrology. Diesbach, Berlin, pp 133–140

Sommer L (2001) Context-dependent regulation of fate decisions in multipotent progenitor cells of the peripheral nervous system. Cell Tissue Res 305:211–216

Song H-j, Stevens CF, Gage FH (2002) Neural stem cells from adult hippocampus develop essential properties of functional CNS neurons. Nat Neurosci 5:438–445

Stocco DM (2007) The role of StAR in Leydig cell steroidogenesis. In: Payne AH, Hardy MP (eds) Contemporarry endocrinology: the Leydig cell in health and disease. Humana, Totowa, pp 149–155

Sugiyama T, Kohara H, Noda M, Nagasawa T (2006) Maintenance of the hematopoietic stem cell pool by CXCL12-CXCR4 chemokine signaling in bone marrow stromal cell nishes. Immunity 25:977–988

Sun Y, Jin K, Xie L, Childs J, Mao XO, Logvinova A, Greenberg DA (2003) VEGF-induced neuroprotection, neurogenesis, and angiogenesis after focal cerebral ischemia. J Clin Invest 111:1843–1851

Suwińska A, Czołowska R, O d e ski W, Tarkowski AK (2008) Blastomeres of the mouse embryo lose totipotency after the fifth cleavage division: expression of Cdx2 and Oct4 and developmental potential of inner and outer blastomeres of 16- and 32-cell embryos. Dev Biol 322:133–144

Suzuki M, Wright LS, Marwah P, Lardy HA, Svendsen CN (2004) Mitotic and neurogenic effects of dehydroepiandrosterone (DHEA) on human neural stem cell cultures derived from the fetal cortex. Proc Natl Acad Sci USA 101:3202–3207

Suzuki T, Nishiama K, Murayama S, Yamamoto A, Sato S, Kanazawa I, Sakaki Y (1996) Regional and cellular presenilin 1 gene expression in human and rat tissues. Biochem Biophys Res Comm 219:708–713

Swredloff RS, Wang C (2007) Clinical evaluation of Leydig cell function. In: Payne AH, Hardy MP (eds) Contemporarry endocrinology: the Leydig cell in health and disease. Humana, Totowa, pp 443–458

Syder AJ, Karam SM, Mills JC, Ippolito JE, Ansari HR, Farook V, Gordon JI (2004) A transgenic mouse model of metastatic carcinoma involving transdifferentiation of a gastric epithelial lineage progenitor to a neuroendocrine phenotype. Proc Natl Acad Sci USA 101:4471–4476

Takahashi Y, Kitadai Y, Bucana CD, Cleary KR, Ellis LM (1995) Expression of vascular endothelial growth factor and its receptor, KDR, correlates with vascularity, metastasis, and proliferation of human colon cancer. Cancer Res 55:3964–3968

Tam PP, Snow MH (1981) Proliferation and migration of primordial germ cells during compensatory growth in mouse embryos. J Embryol Exp Morphol 64:133–147

Tamaki T, Akatsuka A, Ando K, Nakamura Y, Matsizawa H, Hotta T, Roy RR, Edgerton VR (2002) Identification of myogenic-endothelial progenitor cells in the interstitial spaces of skeletal muscle. J Cell Biol 157:571–577

Tamaki T, Akatsuka A, Okada Y, Matsuzaki Y, Okano H, Kimura M (2003) Growth and differentiation potential of main- and side-population cells derived from murine skeletal muscle. Exp Cell Res 291:83–90

Tamaki T, Uchiyama Y, Okada Y, Ishikawa T, Sato M, Akatsuka A, Asahara T (2005) Functional recovery of damaged skeletal muscle through synchronized vasculogenesis, myogenesis, and neurogenesis by muscle-derived stem cells. Circulation 112:2857–2866

Tamamaki N, Nakamura K, Okamoto K, Kaneko T (2001) Radial glia is a progenitor of neocortical neurons in the developing cerebral cortex. Neurosci Res 41:51–60

Tan KAL, De Gendt K, Atanassova N, Walker M, Sharpe RM, Saunders PTK, Denolet E, Verhoeven G (2005) The role of androgens in Sertoli cell proliferation and functional maturation: studies in mice with total or Sertoli cell-selective ablation of the androgen receptor. Endocrinology 146:2674–2683

Tang H, Brennan J, Karl J, Hamada Y, Raetzman L, Capel B (2008) Notch signalling maintains Leydig progenitor cells in the mouse testis. Development 135:3745–3753

Tavian M, Zheng B, Oberlin E, Crisan M, Sun B, Huard J, Péault B (2005) The vascular wall as a source of stem cells. Ann N Y Acad Sci 1044:41–50

Teerds K (1996) Regeneration of Leydig cells after depletion by EDS: a model for postnatal Leydig cell regeneration. In: Payne AH, Hardy MP, Russel LD (eds) The Leydig cell. Cache River, Vienna, pp 203–219

Teerds KJ, Rijntjes E (2007) Dynamics of Leydig cell regeneration after EDS. A model for postnatal Leydig cell development. In: Payne AH, Hardy MP (eds) Contemporarry endocrinology: the Leydig cell in health and disease. Humana, Totowa, pp 91–116

Teerds KJ, de Boer-Brower M, Dorrington JH, Balvers M, Ivell R (1999) Identification of markers for precursor and Leydig cell differentiation in adult rat testis following ethane dimethyl sulphonate administration. Biol Reprod 60:1437–1445

Teerds KJ, Rijntjes E, Veldhuizen-Tsoerkan MB, Rommerts FFG, de Boer-Brouwer M (2007) The development of rat Leydig cell progenitors in vitro: how essential is luteinizing hormone? J Endocrinol 194:579–593

Theise ND, Saxena R, Portmann BC, Thung SN, Yee H, Ghiriboga L, Kumar A, Crawford JM (1999) The canals of Hering and hepatic stem cells in humans. Hepathology 30:1425–1433

Thomas S, Vanuystel J, Grudel G, Rodriguez V, Burt D, Gnudi L, Hartley B, Viberti G (2000) Vascular endothelial growth factor receptors in human mesangium in vitro and in glomerular disease. J Am Soc Nephrol 11:1236–1243

Thomas WE (1999) Brain macrophages: on the role of pericytes and perivascular cells. Brain Res Rev 31:42–57

Tijmes M, Pedraza R, Valladares L (1996) Melatonin in the rat testis: evidence for local synthesis. Steroids 61:65–68

Tilmann C, Capel B (1999) Mesonephric cell migration induces testis cord formation and Sertoli cell differentiation in the mammalian gonad. Development 126:2883–2890

Tilmann C, Capel B (2002) Cellular and molecular pathways regulating mammalian sex determination. Recent Prog Horm Res 57:1–18

Tillmanns J, Rota M, Hosoda T, Misao T, Esposito G, Gonzalez A, Vitale S, Parolin C, Yasizawa-Amano S, Muraski J, De Angelis A, LeCapitaine N, Siggins RW, Loredo M, Bearzi C, Bolli R, Urbanek K, Leri A, Kajstura J, Anversa P (2008) Formation of large coronary arteries by cardiac progenitor cells. Proc Natl Acad Sci USA 105:1668–1673

Tinajero JC, Fabbri A, Dufau ML (1993a) Serotonergic inhibition of rat Leydig cell function by propanolol. Endocrinology 133:257–264

Tinajero JC, Fabbri A, Ciocca DR, Dufau ML (1993b) Serotonin secretion from rat Leydig cells. Endocrinology 133:3026–3029

Toma JG, Akhavan M, Fernandes KJL, Barnabé-Heider F, Sadikot A, Kaplan DR, Miller FD (2001) Isolation of multipotent adult stem cells from the dermis of mammalian skin. Nat Cell Biol 3:778–784

Tomita Y, Matsomura K, Wakamatsu Y, Matsuzaki Y, Shibuya I, Kawaguchi H, Ieda M, Kanakubo S, Shimazaki T, Ogawa S, Osumi N, Okano H, Fukuda K (2005) Cardiac neural crest cells contribute to the dormant multipotent stem cell in the mammalian heart. J Cell Biol 26:1135–1146

Tondreau T, Lagneaux L, Dejeneffe M, Massy M, Mortier C, Delforge A, Bron D (2004) Bone marrow-derived mesenchymal stem cells already express specific neural proteins before any differentiation. Differentiation 72:319–326

Tondreau T, Dejeneffe M, Meuleman N, Stamatopoulos B, Delforge A, Martiat P, Bron D, Lagneaux L (2008) Gene expression pattern of functional neuronal cells derived from human bone marrow mesenchymal stromal cells. BMC Genomics 9:166.doi:10.1186/1471-2164-9-166

Tong MH, Christenson LK, Song W-C (2004) Aberrant cholesterol transport and impaired steroidogenesis in Leydig cells lacking estrogen sulfotransferase. Endocrinology 145:2487–2497

Torrente Y, Tremblay J-P, Pisati F, Belicchi M, Rossi B, Sironi M, Fortunato F, El Fahime M, D'Angelo MG, Caron NJ, Constantin G, Paulin D, Scarlato G, Bresolin N (2001) Intraarterial injection of muscle-derived CD34+Sca-1+ stem cells restores systrophin in mdx mice. J Cell Biol 152:335–348

Towler DA (2003) Angiogenesis and marrow stromal cell fates: roles in bone strength. Osteoporos Int 14(Suppl 5):S46–S53

Trainor PA, Melton KR, Manzanares M (2003) Origins and plasticity of neural crest cells and their roles in jaw and craniofacial evolution. Int J Dev Biol 47:541–553

Treutelaar MK, Skidmore JM, Dias-Leme CL, Hara M, Zhang L, Simeone D, Martin DM, Burant CF (2003) Nestin-lineage cells contribute to the microvasculature but not endocrine cells of the islet. Diabetes 52:2503–2512

Tropel P, Platet N, Platel J-C, No l D, Albrieux M, Benabid A-L, Berger F (2006) Functional neuronal differentiation of bone marrow-derived mesenchymal stem cells. Stem Cells 24:2868–2876

Tsong SD, Phillips D, Halmi N, Liotta AS, Margioris A, Bardin CW, Krieger DT (1982) ACTH- and beta-endorphin-related peptides are present in multiple sites in the reproductive tract of male rat. Endocrinology 110:2204–2206

Turnbull AV, Rivier C (1997) Inhibition of gonadotropin-induced testosterone secretion by the intracerebroventricular injection of interleukin-1ß in the male rat. Endocrinology 138:1008–1013

Turner DL, Cepko CL (1987) A common progenitor for neurons and glia persists in rat retina late in development. Nature 328:131–136

Tyler-McMahon BM, Boules M, Richelson E (2000) Neurotensin: peptide for the next millenium. Regul Peptides 93:125–136

Ungefroren H, Davidoff M, Ivell R (1994) Post-translational block in oxytocin gene expression within the seminiferous tubules of the bovine testis. J Endocrinol 140:63–72

Vaittinen S, Lukka R, Sahlgren C, Rantanen J, Hurme T, Lendahl U, Eriksson JE, Kalimo H (1999) Specific and innervation-regulated expression of the intermediate filament protein nestin at neuromuscular and myotendinous junctions in skeletal muscle. Am J Pathol 154:591–600

Vaittinen S, Lukka R, Sahlgren C, Hurme, Rantanen J, Lendahl U, Eriksson JE, Kalimo H (2001) The expression of intermediate filament protein nestin as related to vimentin and desmin in regenerating skeletal muscle. J Neuropath Exp Neurol 60:588–597

Valenti S, Guido R, Guisti M, Giordano G (1995) In vitro acute and prolonged effects on purified Leydig cell steroidogenesis and adenosine-3',5'-monophosphate production. Endocrinology 136:5357–5362

Van Voorhis BJ, Dunn MS, Snyder GD, Weiner CP (1994) Nitric oxide: an autocrine regulator of human granulosa-luteal cell steroidogenesis. Endocrinology 135:1799–1806

Vera H, Tijmes M, Ronco AM, Valladares LE (1993) Melatonin binding sites in interstitial cells from immature rat testes. Biol Res 26:337–340

Vergouwen RP, Jacobs SG, Huiskamp R, Davids JA, de Rooij DG (1991) Proliferative activity of gonocytes, Sertoli cells and interstitial cells during testicular development in mice. J Reprod Fertil 93:233–243

Verhoeven G, Cailleau J (1987) A Leydig cell stimulatory factor produced by human testicular tubules. Mol Cell Endocrinol 49:2204–2206

Vescovi A, Gritti A, Cossu G, Galli R (2002) Neural stem cells: plasticity and their transdifferentiation potential. Cell Tissue Organs 171:64–78

Vidal VP, Chaboissier M-C, de Rooij DG, Schedl A (2001) Sox9 induces testis development in XX transgenic mice. Nat Genet 28:216–217

Vincent J-P, Mazella J, Kitabgi P (1999) Neurotensin and neurotensin receptors. Trends Pharmacol Sci 20:302–309

von Ebner V (1871) Untersuchungen über den Bau der Samenkanälchen und die Entwicklung der Spermatozoiden bei den Säugetieren und beim Menschen. Rollets Unters Inst Physiol Histol Graz 2:200–215235-236

von Ebner V (1902) A. Koelliker's Handbuch der Gewebelehre des Menschen, 6th edn. Engelmann, Leipzig

von Lenhossèk M (1897) Beiträge zur Kenntniss der Zwischenzellen des Hodens. Arch Anat Phys Anat Abt 65-85 von Hansemann D (1895) Über die sogenannten Zwischenzellen des Hodens und deren Bedeutung bei pathologischen Veränderungen. Virchows Arch A 142:538–546

von Mihalkowics VG (1873) Beiträge zur Anatomie und Histologie des Hodens. Sbr Kgl Sachs Gesell Wiss Leipzig 25:367

Vornberger W, Prins G, Musto NA, Suarez-Quian CA (1994) Androgen receptor distribution in rat testis: new implications for androgen regulation of spermatogenesis. Endocrinology 134:2307–2316

Wakui S, Yokoo K, Muto T, Suzuki Y, Takahashi H, Furusato M, Hano H, Endou H, Kanai Y (2006) Localization of Ang-1, -2, Tie-2, and VEGF expression at endothelial-pericyte interdigitation in rat angiogenesis. Lab Invest 86:1172–1184

Waldeyer W (1870) Über Bindegewebszellen. Archiv Mikrosk Anat 11:176–194

Waldeyer W (1872) Die Entwicklung der Carcinome. Virchows Archiv 55:67–159

Wang S, Bray P, McCaffrey T, March K, Hempstead BL, Kraemer R (2000) p75NTR mediates neurotropin-induced apoptosis of vascular smooth muscle cells. Am J Pathol 157:1247–1258

Wang X, Al-Dhalimy, Lagasse E, Finegold M, Grompe M (2001) Liver repopulation and correction of metabolic liver disease by transplanted adult mouse pancreatic cells. Am J Pathol 158:571–579

Wang X, Foster M, Al-Dhalimy M, Lagasse E, Finegold M, Grompe M (2003) The origin and liver repopulating capacity of murine oval cells. Proc Natl Acad Sci USA 100:11881–11888

Wang Y, Goligorsky MS, Lin M, Wilcox JN, Marsden PA (1997) A novel, testis-specific mRNA transcript encoding NH2-terminal truncated nitric-oxide synthase. J Biol Chem 272:11392–11401

Wang Y, Newton DC, Miller TL, Teichert A-M, Phillips MJ, Davidoff MS, Marsden PA (2002) An alternative promoter of the human neuronal nitric oxide synthase gene is expressed specifically in Leydig cells. Am J Pathol 160:369–380

Wasteson P, Johansson BR, Jukkola T, Breuer S, Akyürek LM, Partinen J, Lindahl P (2008) Developmental origin of smooth muscle cells in the descending aorta in mice. Development 135:1823–1832

Waters JM, Richardson GD, Jahoda CAB (2007) Hair follicle stem cells. Semin Cell Dev Biol 18:245–254

Wattenberg LW (1958) Microscopic histochemical demonstration of steroid-3ß-ol-dehydrogenase in tissue sections. J Histochem Cytochem 6:225–232

Watzka M (1955) Die Leydigschen Zwischenzellen im Funiculus spermaticus des Menschen. Z Zellforsch Mikrosk Anat 43:206–213

Weber DS (2008) A novel mechanism of vascular smooth muscle cell regulation by Notch: platelet-derived growth factor receptor-2 expression? Circ Res 102:1448–1450

Weerasooriya TR, Yamamoto T (1985) Three-dimensional organisation of the vasculature of the rat spermatic cord and testis. A scanning electron-microscopic study of vascular corrosion casts. Cell Tissue Res 241:317–323

Weinbauer CF, Nieschlag E (1990) The role of testosterone in spermatogenesis, In: Nieschlag E, Behre HM (eds) Testosterone: action, deficiency, substitution. Springer, Berlin, pp 23–50

Weinbauer GF, Nieschlag E (1995) Gonadotrophin control of testicular germ cell development. In: Mukhopadhyay AK Raizada MK (eds) Tissue renin-angiotensin systems. Current concepts of local regulators in reproductive and endocrine organs. Plenum, New York, pp 55–65

Weinstein BM (2005) Vessels and nerves: marching to the same tune. Cell 120:299–302

Weissman BA, Niu E, Ge R, Sottas CM, Holmes M, Hutson JC, Hardy MP (2005) Paracrine modulation of androgen synthesis in rat Leydig cells by nitric oxide. J Androl 26:369–378

Weissman IL (2000) Stem cells: units of development, units of regeneration, and units in evolution. Cell 100:157–168

Weissman IL, Anderson DJ, Gage F (2001) Stem and progenitor cells: origins, phenotypes, lineage commitments, and transdifferentiation. Annu Rev Cell Dev Biol 17:387–403

Welch C, Watson ME, Poth M, Hong T, Francis GL (1995) Evidence to suggest nitric oxide is an interstitial regulator of Leydig cell steroidogenesis. Metabolism 44:234–238

Wen PH, Friedrich VL Jr, Shioi J, Robakis NK, Elder GA (2002) Presenilin-1 is expressed in neural progenitor cells in the hippocampus of adult mice. Neurosci Lett 318:53–56

Wen PH, De Gasperi R, Sosa MAG, Rocher AB, Friedrich VL Jr, Hof PR, Elder GA (2005) Selective expression of presenilin 1 in neural progenitor cells rescues the cerebral hemorrhages and cortical lamination defects in presenilin 1-null mutant mice. Development 132:3873–3883

Weng Q, Medan MS, Watanabe G, Tsubota T, Tanioka Y, Taya K (2005) Immunolocalization of steroidogenic enzymes P450scc, 3ßHSD, P450c17, and Pr50arom in Göttingen miniature pig testes. J Reprod Dev 51:299–304

Whitehead RH (1904) The embryonic development of the interstitial cells of Leydig. Am J Anat 3:167–182

Wiese C, Rolletschek A, Kania G, Blyszezuk P, Tarasov KV, Tarasova Y, Wersto RP, Boheler KR, Wobus AM (2004) Nestin expression – a property of multi-lineage progenitor cells? Cell Mol Life Sci 61:2510–2522

Wilber JF, Feng P, Li Q-L, Shi ZX (1996) The thyrotropin-releasing hormone gene. Differential regulation, expression, and function in hypothalamus and two unexpected extra-hypotlialamic loci, the heart and testis. Trends Endocrinol Metab 7:93–100

Wilhelm D, Martinson F, Bradford S, Wilson MJ, Combes AN, Beverdam A, Bowles J, Mizusaki H, Koopman P (2005) Sertoli cell differentiation is induced both cell-autonomously and trough prostaglandin signaling during mammalaian sex determination. Dev Biol 287:111–124

Wilhelm D, Palmer S, Koopman P (2007) Sex determination and gonadal development in mammals. Physiol Rev 87:1–28

Wilson MJ, Bowles J, Koopman P (2006) The matricellular protein SPARC is internalized in Sertoli, Leydig, and germ cells during testis differentiation. Mol Reprod Dev 73:531–539

Woodbury D, Reynolds K, Black IB (2002) Adult bone marrow stem cells express germline, ectodermal, endodermal, and mesodermal genes prior to neurogenesis. J Neurosci Res 96:908–917

Wright E, Hargrave MR, Christiansen J, Cooper L, Kum J, Evans T, Gangadharan U, Greenfeld A, Koopman R (1995) The Sry-related gene Sox9 is expressed during chondrogenesis in mouse embryos. Nat Genet 9:15–20

Wulf GG, Luo K-L, Jackson KA, Brenner MK, Goodell MA (2003) Cells of the hepatic side population contribute to liver regeneration and can be replenished by bone marrow stem cells. Haematologia 88:368–378

Yamada Y, Takakura N (2006) Physiological pathway of differentiation of hematopoietic stem cell population into mural cells. J Exp Med 203:1055–1065

Yamaguchi F, Yamaguchi K, Tokuda M (2000) Presenilin-1 protein specifically expressed in Leydig cells with its expression level increased during rat testis development. Int J Biochem Cell Biol 32:81–87

Yamashima T, Tonchev AB, Vachkov IH, Popivanova BK, Seki T, Sawamoto K, Okano H (2004) Vascular adventitia generates neuronal progenitors in the monkey hippocampus after ischemia. Hippocampus 14:861–875

Yamashita J, Itoh H, Hirashima M, Ogawa M, Nishikawa S, Yurugi T, Nalto M, Nakao K, Nishikawa S-I (2000) Flk1-positive cells derived from embryonic stem cells serve as vascular progenitors. Nature 408:92–96

Yamauchi Y, Abe K, Mantani A, Hitoshi Y, Suzuki M, Osuzu F, Kuratani S, Yamamura K-I (1999) A novel technique that allows specific marking of the neural crest cell lineage in mice. Dev Biol 212:191–203

Yamazaki Y, Mann MRW, Lee SS, Marh J, McCarrey JR, Yanagomachi R, Bartolomei MS (2003) Reprogramming of primordial germ cells begins before migration into the genital ridge, making these cells inadequate donors for reproductive cloning. Proc Natl Acad Sci USA 100:12207–12212

Yan W, Kero J, Huhtaniemi I, Toppari J (2000) Stem cell factor functions as survival factor for mature Leydig cells and a growth factor for precursor Leydig cells after ethylene dimethane sulfonate treatment: implication of a role of the stem cell factor/c-kit system in Leydig cell development. Dev Biol 227:169–182

Yang L, Li S, Hatch H, Ahrens K, Cornelius JG, Petersen BE, Peck AB (2002) In vitro trans-differentiation of adult hepatic stem cells into pancreatic endocrine hormone-producing cells. Proc Natl Acad Sci USA 99:8078–8083

Yang ZW, Kong LS, Guo Y, Yin JQ, Mills N (2006) Histological changes of the testis and epididymis in adult rats as a result of Leydig cell destruction after ethane dimethane sulfonate treatment: a morphometric study. Asian J Androl 8:289–299

Yao HH-C, Barsoum I (2007) Fetal Leydig cells. Origin, regulation, and function. In: Payne AH, Hardy MP (eds) Contemporarry endocrinology: the Leydig cell in health and disease. Humana, Totowa, pp 47–54

Yao HH-C, Capel B (2002) Disruption of testis cords by cyclopamine or forskolin reveals independent cellular pathways in testis organogenesis. Dev Biol 246:356–365

Yao HH-C, Whoriskey W, Capel B (2002) Desert Hedgehog/Patched 1 signaling specifies fetal Leydig cell fate in testis organogenesis. Genes Dev 16:1433–1440

Yao HH-C, Matzuk MM, Jorgez CJ, Menke DB, Page DC, Swain A, Capel B (2004) Follistatin operates downstream of Wnt4 in mammalian ovary organogenesis. Dev Dyn 230:210–215

Yao HH-C, Aardema J, Holthusen K (2006) Sexually dimorphic regulation of inhibin B in establishing gonatal vasculature in mice. Biol Reprod 74:978–983

Yazawa T, Mizutani T, Yamada K, Kawata H, Sekiguchi T, Yoshino M, Kajitani T, Shou Z, Umezawa A, Miyamoto K (2006) Differentiation of adult stem cells derived from bone marrow stroma into Leydig and adrenocortical cells. Endocrinology 147:4104–4111

Yoder MC, Hiatt K, Dutt P, Mukherjee P, Bodine DM, Orlic D (1997) Characterization of definitive lymphohematopoietic stem cells in the day 9 murine yolk sac. Immunity 7:335–344

Young HM (2004) Existence of reserve quiescent stem cells in adults, from amphibians to humans. Curr Top Microbiol Immunol 280:71–109

Yovchev MI, Grozdanov PN, Zhou H, Racherla H, Guha C, Dabeva MD (2008) Identification of adult hepatic progenitor cells capable of repopulating injured rat liver. Histopathology 47:636–647

Yu H, Fang D, Kumar SM, Li L, Nguyen TK, Acs G, Herlyn M, Xu X (2006) Isolation of a novel population of multipotent adult stem cells from human hair follicles. Am J Pathol 168:1879–1888

Zagon IS, Rhodes RE, McLaughlin PJ (1986) Localization of enkephalin immunoreactivity in diverse tissues and cells of the developing and adult rat. Cell Tissue Res 246:561–565

Zammit PS, Partridge TA, Yablonka-Reuveni Z (2006) The skeletal muscle satellite cell: the stem cell that came in from the cold. J Histochem Cytochem 54:1177–1191

Zannettino ACW, Paton S, Arthur A, Khor F, Itescu S, Gimble JM, Gronthos S (2007a) Multipotential human adipose-derived stromal stem cells exhibit a perivascular phenotype in vitro and in vivo. J Cell Physiol 214:413–421

Zannettino ACW, Paton S, Kortesidis A, Khor F, Itescu S, Gonthos S (2007b) Human multipotential mesenchymal/stromal stem cells are derived from a discrete subpopulation of STRO-1bright/CD34-/Cd45-/glycophorin-A-bone marrow cells. Haematologica 92:1707–1708

Zengin E, Chalajour F, Gehling UM, Ito WD, Treede WD, Lauke H, Weil J, Reichenspurner H, Kilic N, Ergün S (2006) Vascular wall resident progenitor cells: a source for postnatal vasculogenesis. Development 133:1543–1551

Zhang H, Vutskits L, Pepper MS, Kiss JZ (2003) VEGF is a chemoattractant for FGF-2-stimulated neural progenitors. J Cell Biol 22:1375–1384

Zhang S-H, Zhang Y-Q, Vacca-Galloway LL (1995) Identification of thyrotropin-releasing hormone receptor mRNA in the Leydig cells of the mouse testis by in situ hybridization. Neuropeptides 29:309–313

Zhang Y, Ge R, Hardy MP (2008) Androgen-forming Leydig cells: identification, function and therapeutic potential. Dis Markers 24:277–286

Zhao C, Deng W, Gage FH (2008) Mechanisms and functional implications of adult neurogenesis. Cell 132:645–660

Zhu Y, Jin K, Mao XO, Greenberg DA (2003) Vascular endothelial growth factor promotes proliferation of cortical neuron precursors by regulating E2F expression. FASEB J 17:186–193

Zimmerman L, Lendahl U, Cunningham M, McKay R, Parr B, Gavin B, Mann J, Vassileva G, McMahon A (1994) Independent regulatory elements in the nestin gene direct transgene expression to neural stem cells or muscle precursors. Neuron 12:11–24

Zimmermann K (1923) Der feinere Bau der Blutkapillaren. Z Anat Entwicklungsgesch 68:29–109

Zulewski H, Abraham EJ, Gerlach MJ, Daniel PB, Moritz W, Müller B, Vallejo M, Thomas MK, Habener JF (2001) Multipotential nestin-positive stem cells isolated from adult pancreatic islets differentiate ex vivo into pancreatic endocrine, exocrine, and hepatic phenotypes. Diabetes 50:521–533

Subject Index

A
AADC 34
A2B5 40, 65
acetylcholine 30, 32
activin 23, 91
adipocytes 65, 73, 76, 80, 100
adult stem cells 52, 73, 79, 80, 97, 98
adult-type 27, 49, 50, 69, 82–85
AGM region 93, 94, 102, 103
aminopeptidase A 71, 79
aminopeptidase N 71, 79
ancestor 83, 90, 97, 99, 101, 102, 106
androgens 1, 25, 6, 19–21, 23, 32, 86
androgen receptors 20, 86
ANGPT1 42
ANGPT2 41
Angiopoietin1,2 41, 42, 72
angiotensin I 40
angiotensin II 24, 41
angiotensin-converting enzyme 40
angiotensin receptor I 41
ANP 39
aorta 79, 92, 93, 101, 102, 106
apoptosis 21, 32, 34, 54, 59
arginine-vasopressin 23
aromatase 19, 32

B
basement membrane 67, 68, 70, 95, 106
BDNF 34
BNP 39
branching processes 17
BrdU 54, 58–61, 83

C
calcitonin 23
calcitonin gene-related peptide 32
CaM 31, 32
Ca^{2+}/CaM PK II 31, 32
cardiac mesenchymal stem cells 77
catecholamines 23, 34
cGMP 25, 31–33, 39
CNP 39
CNPase 40
Co-cells 11, 36
compartmentalizing cells 14, 15, 36
connexin 43 15
CRH 23, 36
chromogranin A 8
CytP450scc 29, 36, 56, 58, 61–63, 65, 66, 85, 86, 89, 95

D
DBH 34
DHEA 21
dental pulp 6, 76
desmosome 14
development 75, 78, 80–87, 90–103, 105, 106
 - fetal 5, 52
 - normal 84, 85
 - postnatal 50, 51, 53, 54, 84, 85, 87, 89, 95–97
 - prenatal 49, 63
dormant 2, 52, 53, 100

E
ectoderm(-al) 45, 51, 64, 75, 90, 98, 100, 106
EDS 50–62, 64–69, 71, 79, 83, 84, 87
EGF 23, 38
EG-VEGF 41
electron microscopy 7, 13
embryonic stem cells 72, 74, 97
endoderm(-al) 51, 64, 78, 90, 106
endothelial cells 34, 41, 42, 47, 50, 67, 69–72, 74–81, 92, 93
endothelins 23
environmental influences 28
epiblast 1, 45, 51, 52, 73, 97, 100, 106
epigenetic factors 64, 94

F
fetal stem cells 52
fetal-type 52, 53, 56, 58, 59, 61, 67, 69, 83–85, 87, 89, 95
FGF2 23, 41, 42, 65, 69, 71, 83
FGF9 47, 48
Fibroblasts 50, 63, 65, 72, 73, 77, 80, 87, 98
FSH 23, 30

G
3G5 71, 76, 78
GABA 30, 31
GABA-A receptors 31
GalC 40
gap junctions 14, 15, 18, 70, 72
germ cells 1, 5, 30, 32, 45, 46, 47, 59, 68, 103
glia (glial) cells 1, 2, 7, 11, 26, 28, 36, 40, 52, 58, 62, 63, 65, 67, 69, 70, 74, 75, 80, 81, 83, 86, 98–100
  - astrocytes 27, 28, 40, 72, 74, 8
  - oligodendrocytes 40, 74
  - radial 80, 99
GDNF 34, 65, 83
GFRα-1 34, 65
GFRα-2 34, 65
GFAP 40, 57, 65, 74, 75, 99, 100
glycocorticoids 23
GHRH 36
GnRH 24, 36
gonad 43, 45–48, 52, 89–94, 102, 103
green fluorescent protein 58, 66
GUCY1B3 41
guinea pig 27, 28, 32

H
hamster 28, 38, 40, 53, 54, 98
heart 39, 52, 77
hCG 6, 20, 33, 36
hematopoietic 52, 64, 73–79, 93, 103
heterogenous 76
HGF 72
histochemistry 6
human 19, 73, 102
  - adipose tissue 78, 79
  - bone marrow 76, 100
  - brain 38, 39, 74
  - chorionic gonadotropin 6, 20, 33, 86
  - embryos 41, 87, 101
  - heart 39
  - kidney 75
  - Leydig cells 9–13, 15–18, 29, 35, 39

  - liver 39
  - macrophages 32
  - pancreas 75
  - spleen 39
  - stem cells 78
  - testis 9, 10, 14, 15, 37, 66, 87
  - ureter 30
hypoblast 51
5-HT 23, 32, 38
hypothalamus 1, 6. 20
hypophysis 20
3β-HSD 20, 84, 86

I
immunohistochemistry 27, 35, 39, 40, 53, 58, 75,
inhibin 23, 91
interleukin-1 23, 26, 30, 43
interstitium 47, 50, 63, 86, 107
intertubular space 85, 87

K
Kidney 39, 75, 76, 79

L
LacZ 72, 92, 102
Leydig cells
  - adult 8, 49, 50, 53, 54, 63, 67, 82, 89
  - blast 2, 8, 50, 60, 65, 83
  - endocrine 1, 5, 19
  - fetal 87, 89, 91, 99, 100, 106
  - immature 15, 30, 49, 58, 59, 63, 86, 87, 101
  - mature 19, 21, 49, 58, 59, 86, 87
  - neonatal 15
  - neuroendocrine 6, 23, 49, 50, 53, 65
  - progenitors 50, 53, 55, 56, 66, 79, 86, 99
  - stem/progenitor 27, 53, 59, 60, 82, 98
  - young 87, 105, 106
LH 6, 20, 30, 32, 43, 84, 86
LHR 28
LH/hCG receptors 6, 20
LHRH 32
local factors 77, 86
low proliferating 53

M
macrophages 31, 32, 50, 54
MAP-2 27
melatonin 23, 38

Subject Index

mesectoderm 90, 99, 106
mesenchymal cells 36, 43, 60, 67, 90, 101
mesenchymal-neural cells 99–101, 106
mesenchymal stem/stromal cells 64, 73, 77
mesoderm(-al) 51, 64, 73, 76, 80, 90, 98, 102, 106
mesonephric cells 47, 48, 93
microvasculature 59, 70
microcirculation 75
Met-Enk 6, 7
morphology 9–11, 13, 52, 91
mouse 53, 102
multipotent 27, 46, 52, 64, 73, 78, 101
myofibroblasts 33, 42, 47, 64, 101

N

natriuretic peptides 23, 38
NCAM 41, 54, 65, 69, 74
nervous system 7, 27, 39, 56, 74, 95, 99
 - central 27, 30, 41, 52
 - peripheral 11, 33, 39, 52, 79, 100
NG2 54, 60, 72, 83, 99, 101
NGF 33, 34
nestin 38, 39, 50, 56, 58, 60, 61, 66, 83, 101
neural stem cells 2, 21, 52, 74, 81, 98
neuroendocrine cells 27, 33, 40, 43, 62, 67
 - neuroectodermal 7, 53, 79, 79, 80, 90, 98, 106
 - neural crest 53, 79, 90, 98
 - properties 53
NeuroD 28, 57, 65
NF-H 39, 57, 65, 66, 71
NF-M 39
NF-L 39
neurofilament ptoteins 39, 66, 99
NPY 30, 31
neuropeptides 1, 7, 28, 33
neurotensin 30
neurotrophins 33, 34, 39
NeuN 27, 100
neurons 23, 27, 36, 41, 56, 74, 99
niche 2, 53, 63, 80, 106
NO 31
NO/cGMP system 31
noradrenaline 32, 34
NOS 30, 32, 33
NOS-1 31, 32, 33
NOS-2 31, 32
NOS-3 31, 32
NSE 23, 27

O

O4 25, 40, 65
oestrogen 19, 21, 23, 32
 - receptors 20, 21
 - sulfotransferase 21
origin of Leydig cells 1, 30
 - mesenchymal 1, 64, 67, 72, 84, 90
 - neuroectodermal 79
 - neural crest 90, 98, 101, 102
oval stem cells 74, 77
oxytocin 23

P

pancreas 52, 64, 75, 79, 90
p75^{NTR} 24, 64, 74
PCR (RT-PCR) 34, 39, 98
PGCs 45, 46
pericytes 8, 59, 63, 67, 70, 71, 73, 98
pituitary 6, 20, 30, 43
PDGF 23, 41, 42
PDGF-A 38, 42
PDGF-B 26, 42
PDGF-BB 42
PDGF-C 42
PDGF-D 42
PDGFR-α 42
PDGFR-β 26, 42
plasticity 27, 52, 76, 78, 101
pluripotent 52, 63, 73, 102, 106
postnatal development 50, 53, 54, 84, 87
PNMT 23, 24
precursors 19, 27, 51
 - cardiac 77
 - endothelial 74
 - epiblast 51
 - Leydig cell 63, 65, 68, 87, 93, 100, 106
 - mesenchymal 78
 - mesenchymal-neural 101
 - multipotent 27
 - myogenic 76
 - neural 28, 38, 81, 82
 - neural crest 101
 - pericyte 72, 92
 - skin-derived 76
presenilin-1 39
progeny 51, 65, 73, 83, 95, 98, 101
prolactin 23
prorenin 26, 40

Q

quiescent 53

R

Reinke cristalloids 10
rats 40, 69
5α-reductase 19, 86
regeneration 8, 27, 36, 54, 67, 95
rennin 26, 40, 41
RGS5 71, 72
rodent testis 84

S

satellite cells 76, 78
seminiferous epithelium 69
αSMA 71, 79, 98, 101
S-100 25, 40
Schwann cells 40, 101
Sertoli cells 5, 20, 30, 46, 70
SF1 47
sGC 25, 31–33
side-population stem cells 97
silencing 8, 53, 65, 94, 100, 106
skeletal muscle 34, 52, 60, 64, 72, 76, 98
skin 52, 64, 75–79, 100
smooth muscle cells 8, 50, 54, 57, 58, 60, 63, 66, 70
Sox9 47, 93
spermatogenesis 9, 14, 20, 21, 34, 58, 82
spermatogonia 46, 59, 97
stem cells 2, 8, 50, 51, 55, 61, 63, 64, 67, 73, 74, 76, 78, 79, 80, 95, 97, 102, 106
 - adult 2, 8, 52, 73
 - bone marrow 61, 103
 - bone marrow stromal 76
 - bone mesenchymal 73
 - cardiac 77
 - dental pulp 76
 - dormant 2
 - embryonal 52, 72, 73
 - endothelial 103, 106
 - fetal 52
 - haematopoietic 73
 - hepatic 73
 - liver 61, 74
 - mesenchymal 2, 51, 60, 64, 77, 97, 106
 - mesenchymal/stromal 78
 - microvascular 58
 - mural 8
 - neural 21, 33, 38, 61, 72, 74, 98
 - neural crest 77, 98, 103
 - neuroepithelial 74
 - skeletal muscle 61, 76
 - skin 76
substance P (SP) 7, 29, 30, 32, 98

SRY (Sry) 43, 45–47, 91, 92
steroid hormones 47, 99
steroidogenic cells 13, 40
substantia nigra 34, 35
superoxide dismutase 26
synaptophysin 66, 74

T

T3 36, 38
tachykinins 28–30
testis 36, 38–41, 45, 49, 53, 60, 70, 84, 87, 91, 92
 - human 14, 15, 34, 37, 39, 40, 41, 66, 87
 - mouse 53
 - rat 33, 36–38, 53, 55,-57, 60, 67, 70, 97
testicular cords 46, 47, 89, 93
testosterone 6, 19–21, 23, 30, 36, 43, 69, 85, 87
TGFα 23, 26, 38
TGFβ 23, 34, 65, 72
Tn-NOS 31
Totipotent 52
TPH 24, 38
TH 24, 35, 38
TR α 38
TRH 36
TrkA 24, 29, 34, 56, 97
Trkb 24, 34, 65, 74
TrkC 24, 34, 65, 74
thyroid hormones 23, 38
transdifferentiation 58, 63, 65, 66, 82, 83, 85, 89, 95, 98, 105

U

Urogenital ridge 46, 93, 103

V

vascular stem cell niche 2, 63, 64, 80, 106
vascular smooth muscle cells 8, 20, 34, 40, 54, 57, 65, 66, 70, 79, 101, 106
very small embryonic-like stem cells 73, 100, 106
vessels 92
VEGF 26, 41, 42, 65, 69, 72, 75, 79, 82
VEGFR-1 26, 41
VEGFR-2 41

W

western blot 28, 34, 39, 40, 53, 58, 98

Printing and Binding: Stürtz GmbH, Würzburg